THE YOGA MAN(UAL)

JEN MURPHY

FOREWORD BY ANDREW TANNER

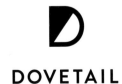

DOVETAIL

CONTENTS

FOREWORD

ANDREW TANNER
CHIEF SPOKESPERSON FOR YOGA ALLIANCE

There are hundreds of yoga books on the market, but only a handful of them are geared toward men. And of those few male-centric yoga guides, most were written by professional wrestlers (such as Diamond Dallas Page) or people who look like professional wrestlers, or are simply a collection of postures for experienced yogis. What has been missing from this conversation is a down-to-earth book that answers the questions men have before they try yoga so they can get the most out of the experience.

This book fills that void. And the fact that it was written by a woman, Jen Murphy, but also includes profiles of a number of men—professional athletes, advanced yogis and regular guys—means it provides the perfect blend of yin and yang. I met Jen two years ago when she interviewed me for her *Wall Street Journal* column. When she asked me to weigh in on the best time to do yoga, I started rambling about some obscure ideas related to circadian rhythms and specific yoga practices for those rhythms. What impressed me about Jen was how she could take what I said and repeat it back to me in a way that was so much simpler and more digestible. Jen is also a woman who really gets guys. This, combined with her expertise as a journalist, athlete, and yoga practitioner, makes her the perfect person to write this book.

As men, when we do something, we like to know how to do it correctly. We don't want to waste time. And, let's face it: we care about what women think. None of us wants to look like a fool in a room full of women in stretchy pants! This well-researched book provides an amazing context for any man thinking of starting to practice yoga. It will help you make well-informed decisions about who to practice yoga with and what style to practice.

In this book you'll read the stories of many different men and their experiences with yoga. From businessmen to athletes to yogis, they generally have the same message: "Yoga is hard and humbling—and so worth it." As the famous stoic philosopher Seneca said, "Difficulties strengthen the mind, as labor does the body." Yoga does both.

Most men would agree that life is a challenge. We all have goals and ideas but often lack the resolve to see them through. What's special about yoga is that once you find the style that works for your body, it cannot do you wrong. Yoga is never a waste of time. Afterward, you will always feel that you're better prepared to tackle life's challenges and more efficiently meet your goals. In my fifteen years of teaching yoga, I've never heard anyone say, "Man, I wish I hadn't taken that class."

If you're feeling lost or just stuck on a plateau in any area of your life, this book can be the gateway to your next great—and rewarding—challenge. I promise that yoga will open up a new world for you. The most important thing I can recommend is that you read this entire book and follow Jen's recommendations on finding teachers and approaches that will work well for you. Yoga is not a one-size-fits-all practice.

I never thought I'd be a yoga teacher, let alone the chief ambassador of the largest yoga association in the world. It took six months of practicing yoga before I was even able to touch my toes—something I hadn't been able to do since childhood. Opening up your body will take time, but it will also open up your mind and allow you to see new opportunities in every moment of your life.

I'm so grateful to Jen for putting this book together and trying to get more men on the mat. As both a man and a yogi, I wholeheartedly endorse this book. At the very least, guys, read this book so you won't look like an ass at the studio.

INTRODUCTION

You're probably wondering why a woman is writing a book about yoga for men. I actually asked the same question when I was approached about the project. Wouldn't a guy know what's best for a guy's mind and body? You could certainly argue that. But this book isn't meant to just tell you how to do yoga; first and foremost, it's intended to convince you to try yoga. And based on the dozens of men I interviewed for this project and the experiences of many of my male friends, I've learned that one of the most common reasons any guy tries yoga is because of a girl. Maybe you want to impress a girl you like, or your girlfriend convinced you (aka forced you) to try it. Perhaps your girlfriend dumped you and you want to heal your broken heart. Or maybe you just want to check out girls stretching in spandex.

Even when the girl part doesn't work out, most guys end up falling in love with the yoga part, and it becomes a relationship they never regret. The hurdle most men have to overcome is that yoga has become one of the few physical activities in which women truly dominate. That can be both humbling and intimidating. My brother, who was a professional bodyboarder in his teens, is a great example. He incorporated yoga into his training so he could safely launch himself off some of the world's most powerful waves, yet he kept his yoga practice a secret. If I ever caught him doing downward dog in his room, he'd threaten to kick my ass if I told anyone at school. Similarly, on snowboarding trips when I was in college, my guy friends would each pull me aside and ask me to show them hip-opening poses—after making me swear I wouldn't tell the others. There's still a stigma that yoga is a "girl thing," when it should actually be viewed as a performance enhancer. Guys shave their legs, adopt fruitarian diets, and lie in float tanks for hours, all to improve their game. Is yoga really more embarrassing than all of that stuff?

The studio can be scary for dudes. You may walk into your first class expecting to score a date, but as soon as you try holding a plank pose for twenty breaths, your libido will go out the window and you'll be cursing the blonde girl in pink tights who pops into handstand every five minutes. No guy wants to look weak in a roomful of girls. And even though yogis insist there is no "good" or "bad" in yoga, it's hard not to notice the girl next to you with her palms flat on the floor in forward fold while your hands are dangling helplessly in front of your very bent knees. It's difficult to embrace the things we suck at. And let's face it, many athletic girls grew up dancing ballet or doing gymnastics, while many boys grew up playing soccer, football, and baseball. We were trained to be flexible; you were trained to be strong. But strength and flexibility are not mutually exclusive, and yoga requires both. Although men and women tend to be at opposite ends of the spectrum, yoga asks everyone to work toward the center.

Developing the courage to do something for yourself, regardless of what it might look like on the outside, is the first step to doing anything, including yoga. And as with any sport or skill, practice makes perfect. You may never master the perfect split or side crow, but that's not the point of yoga. If you practice with some regularity, you'll see incredible gains not just in flexibility, but across all aspects of your life.

I've practiced yoga for more than fifteen years and can honestly say I sucked at it when I started. As a runner and travel writer, I have tight hips and hamstrings from logging countless miles on trails, pavement, and planes. And like many athletes, I have a competitive nature that made yoga a struggle for me. The process of accepting my weaknesses made me become incredibly aware of my body—my muscle imbalances, my tight spots, my breathing, and my focus, or lack thereof. Eventually, I became less concerned with "perfecting" poses and more concerned with how I felt when I was in them. I learned to channel my breath to improve my running and, perhaps more importantly, to manage my day-to-day stress. I have studied yoga around the world and now practice yoga every day, and while my knees still hunch up to my ears in a simple cross-legged seat, my mind is no longer a big to-do list of chatter. I've written the *Wall Street Journal*'s "What's Your Workout?" column for almost thirteen years, and nearly every successful person I've interviewed for that column, male or female, says his or her secret isn't spin class or CrossFit but learning to quiet the mind through yoga.

With this book, I've attempted to demystify yoga so you'll feel more intrigued and excited about it—and less intimidated by it. The following chapters attempt to answer all of the befuddling questions that may cross your mind about yoga, from its origins to many of the newly invented hybrid styles, and from when to practice to what to wear. Hopefully you won't feel as self-conscious visiting a yoga studio once you learn the meaning of terms like *pranayama*, understand basic yoga class etiquette, and know what to do with all of those props. The book also breaks down basic poses and explains the benefits of each so you can string together your own practice for at home, on the road, or even at the office. And just in case you're still dubious about yoga's benefits, I've shared real stories from real guys—professional athletes and desk jockeys, regular practitioners and lapsed yogis. I hope my tips, along with their insights, convince you that yoga isn't just for girls—and that maybe you've been missing out on something awesome.

CHAPTER 1

WHAT YOGA?

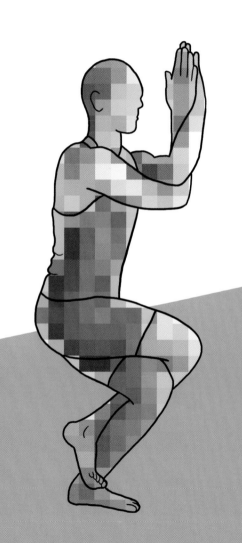

THE ORIGINS OF YOGA

When people think of yoga, they often conjure one of two images: a loincloth-clad old Indian man sitting with his legs behind his head along the Ganges, or a lithe, young Lululemon-dressed yogini sipping kombucha at the studio. This stark contrast underscores the drastic evolution of the practice. What we think of today as a workout for stressed-out women is actually a practice that was created by and for men, popularized by men, and predominantly practiced by men until the past few decades.

The history of yoga remains shrouded in mystery and speculation. Many researchers link its origins to the Indus Valley, where stone carvings depicting people sitting in meditative positions date back some five thousand years. The first written mention of yogic teachings appeared in the Vedas, a collection of Hindu texts from 1200 BCE. These texts include descriptions of mantras, songs, and rituals used by Brahman priests.

Though he wasn't considered a rock star back in the day, the Indian sage Patanjali was, in many ways, the first celebrity yoga guru. The Yoga Sutras, his treatise on yogic philosophy written over two thousand years ago, provides the first real framework for yoga. A collection of 196 aphorisms, the Yoga Sutras are somewhat similar to a modern-day self-help book, instructing practitioners in how to live a more disciplined life by restraining the mind. Yoga, according to Patanjali, "is the restriction of the fluctuations of consciousness" (Sutra 1.2). At that time, yoga was a mental and spiritual practice, not the physical practice we know today. There's no mention of warrior poses or handstands. The only reference to poses in the Yoga Sutras is "a steady and comfortable posture" (Sutra 2.46), referring to the seated postures used for meditation.

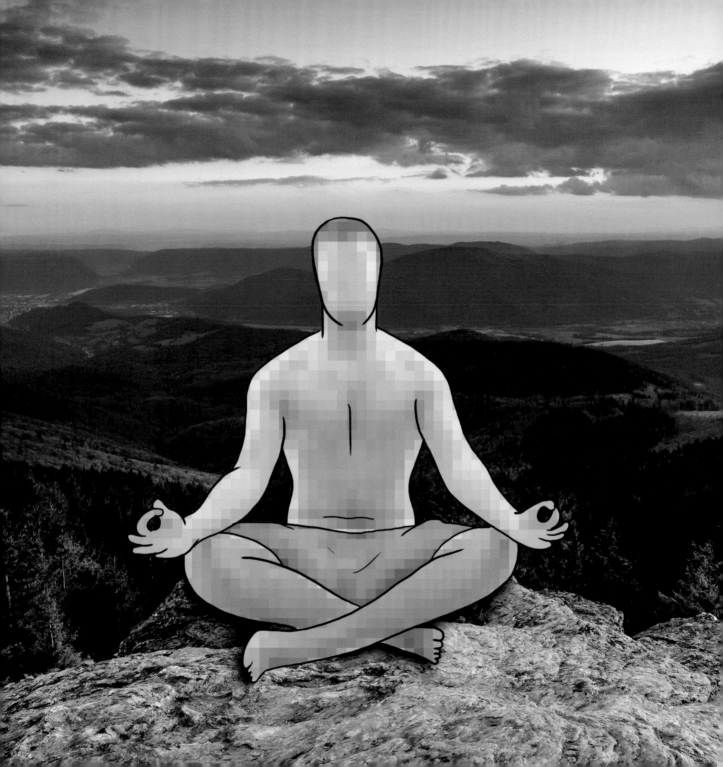

THE EVOLUTION OF OM

The discipline of hatha yoga—the physical practice of yoga that influences most Western styles today—was originally developed to prepare the body and nervous system for stillness, creating the physical stamina needed for meditation. It wasn't until the twentieth century that hatha yoga began to resemble a workout. Yoga guru Tirumalai Krishnamacharya is responsible for putting a CrossFit-style twist on the traditional hatha practice.

Known as the father of modern yoga, Krishnamacharya promoted the vinyasa-style practice of combining movement with the breath and made postures part of meditation rather than just a warm-up for meditation. His practice emphasized therapeutic poses like shoulder stand, as well as flowing sequences such as sun salutation. As the yogi-in-residence at India's Mysore Palace in the 1930s and 1940s, Krishnamacharya was tasked with teaching rambunctious royal boys, which probably explains why he developed a practice that could capture their youthful energy. His fast-flowing style drew from gymnastics, traditional Indian wrestling, and British Army calisthenics. Some of yoga's most influential teachers studied under Krishnamacharya, including his son, T. K. V. Desikachar, as well as B. K. S. Iyengar, K. Pattabhi Jois, and Indra Devi.

These days, yoga students are often warned not to force themselves into poses. That caution perhaps springs from the experiences of B. K. S. Iyengar, who suffered multiple injuries when he followed Krishnamacharya's forceful approach to mastering postures. Iyengar went on to develop his own style of yoga: a slower, alignment-focused practice that utilizes props to help students ease into poses. T. K. V. Desikachar took a more therapeutic approach to the practice and developed what today is known as Viniyoga, a highly individualized style that tailors the practice to each student's specific emotional and physical condition. K. Pattabhi Jois took the opposite approach, embracing Krishnamacharya's energetic practice and creating the dynamic ashtanga style of yoga, which links a precise series of poses with the breath.

YOGA IN AMERICA

You may have noticed that women have had no mention thus far in yoga's history. Yoga was originally a man's world. In the 1890s, American yoga proselytizer Pierre Bernard, known as "the Great Oom," started promoting the tantric yoga philosophy in San Francisco. His open sexual relationships led to yoga becoming associated with sexual promiscuity, and therefore a threat to the purity of American women.

When Russian actress Indra Devi showed up in India to train with Krishnamacharya in the 1930s, he bluntly told her that he didn't teach women. Only begrudgingly, and at the insistence of the maharaja, did he accept her as a student. Today, Devi is often called the First Lady of Yoga and can largely be credited with making the practice not just acceptable, but fashionable for women in America. In 1947, she opened a studio in Hollywood and taught stars like Greta Garbo and Gloria Swanson, and her 1959 book *Yoga for Americans* had housewives across the United States practicing asanas at home.

Walt Baptiste Westernized the practice even further by combining weight training with yoga and meditation. A body-builder and former Mr. America (yes, that was a thing), Baptiste and his wife Magaña opened the first yoga school in San Francisco in 1955 and ushered in the American obsession with power yoga.

Yoga hit the airwaves in the 1960s with American Richard Hittleman's popular TV show *Yoga for Health*. After studying in India, Hittleman had returned to New York and Americanized the practice, introducing a nonreligious style of yoga that emphasized its physical benefits, rather than the spiritual. The approach was a hit with the American mainstream and led to the development of dozens of vigorous new styles.

MODERN-DAY YOGA

Purists may decry yoga's evolution and highly specialized styles like joga (jogging plus yoga), SUP (standup paddleboard) yoga, and even laughter yoga, but that evolution has allowed the benefits of yoga to spread around the globe. Today, more than thirty-seven million Americans do yoga, and ten million of them are men. Yoga has made its way to the offices of Google and Facebook, to public schools and prisons, and even into the training regimens of Olympic and professional athletes. Mark Morrison, the strength and conditioning coach of the Hendrick Motorsports NASCAR racing team, brings in a power yoga teacher because he believes holding poses and incorporating breath work translates into improved focus and judgment on the racetrack. Pete Carroll, head coach of the Seattle Seahawks, introduced meditation and yoga as part of the team's training because he believes happy players are better players. And after the team's 2014 Super Bowl win, his star quarterback, Russell Wilson, credited regular meditation for keeping him relaxed on the field.

In the business world, Stanton Kawer, CEO of Blue Chip Marketing Worldwide, admits he keeps a yoga mat in his car and starts staff meetings by asking everyone to take a deep breath. He says his yoga practice has redefined his expectations for achievement in the office because in yoga, winning isn't about a scorecard; it's about self-mastery. Jim Mulvihill, a cofounder of the Denver-based real estate firm Black Creek Group, says he can't get into the spiritual side of yoga, but he did hire an instructor to work with him and his squash partners so they can avoid typical weekend warrior injuries. Yoga has even found its way to the battlefield through programs like Yoga Warriors International, which provides instruction in calming, hatha-based techniques to active military personnel and veterans suffering from combat stress and post-traumatic stress.

Different people get different things from the practice, whether those benefits are mental, physical, spiritual, or all three. Yoga is no longer a narrowly defined discipline; it's an ever-expanding experience to explore.

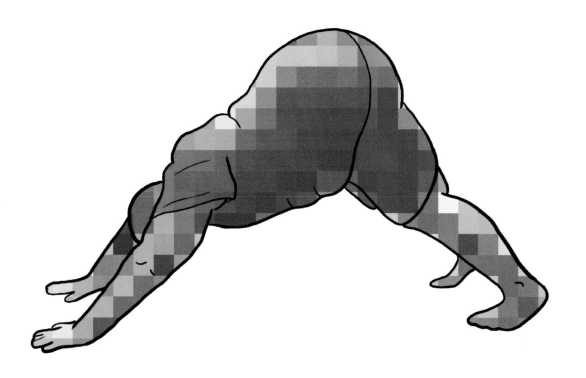

Yoga is for everyone.
No one is too old or too stiff,
too fat or thin or tired.

B.K.S. IYENGAR
FOUNDER OF IYENGAR YOGA

NOTABLE MOMENTS IN YOGA

3000 BCE Stone carvings linked to yoga are created in the Indus Valley.

1200 BCE Yogic teachings are included in the *Vedas*, the oldest known scriptures in the world.

400 BCE The Indian sage Patanjali writes *The Yoga Sutras*, his treatise on yogic philosophy and the first real framework for yoga.

1849 Henry David Thoreau mentions yoga in a letter to his friend H. G. O. Blake, stating "Free in this world as the birds in the air, disengaged from every kind of chains, those who practice the yoga gather in Brahma the certain fruits of their works."

1893 Swami Vivekananda introduces Hinduism to America at the World's Parliament of Religions in Chicago.

1917 The Immigration Act of 1917 restricts Asian-Indians from immigrating to the United States.

1924 Westerners start traveling to the East to seek yoga teachings due to a U.S. quota on Indian immigration.

1947 Indra Devi opens one of the first U.S. yoga studios in Hollywood.

1953 A *Life* magazine story reports that Iyengar yoga is responsible for violinist Yehudi Menuhin's artistic breakthrough.

1955 Walt and Magaña Baptiste open San Francisco's first yoga studio.

1956 Marilyn Monroe tells the media that she practices yoga to improve her legs.

1959 Swami Vishnu-devananda publishes *The Complete Illustrated Book of Yoga*.

1961 Richard Hittleman's *Yoga for Health* becomes the first-ever yoga television series.

1966 B. K. S. Iyengar's *Light on Yoga* is published in the United States, a book that is still considered to be the bible of serious asana practice.

1968 The Beatles travel to India to attend a Transcendental Meditation training session at Maharishi Mahesh Yogi's ashram.

1972 According to Bikram Choudhury, founder of Bikram Yoga, president Richard Nixon came to him for help while suffering from advanced thrombophlebitis in his left leg.

1975 The California Yoga Teachers Association founds *Yoga Journal*.

1976 T. K. V. Desikachar founds the Krishnamacharya Yoga Mandiram, a yoga center in Madras, India focused on yoga's therapeutic benefits.

1979 The Yoga Federation of India holds the first National Yoga Championships.

1987 The Washington, D.C.-based nonprofit organization Yoga Alliance is formed to create minimum standards for yoga teachers.

1998 Lululemon, a yoga-inspired apparel company, is founded in Vancouver by Chip Wilson.

2003 Rajashree Choudhury founds the International Yoga Sports Federation, a governing body for the sport of yoga, in Los Angeles. The IYSF works with other yoga federations to lobby for yoga sports, athletic competitions based on yoga postures, to become an Olympic sport.

2006 Gopi Kallayil joins Google as chief evangelist for brand marketing and introduces yoga and mindfulness programs to the company.

2007 Designer Donna Karan cofounds the Urban Zen initiative, which promotes complementary care, including yoga therapy, for cancer patients.

2011 Broga, a strong, energetic yoga style geared toward men, is cofounded by Adam O'Neill and Robert Sidoti in Massachusetts.

2012 Anusaragate breaks, with celebrity yoga teacher John Friend being accused of a sex scandal.

2012 Former pro wrestler Diamond Dallas Page introduces DDP Yoga, which promises ripped abs and a workout comparable to running, but with no impact.

2013 Seattle Seahawks head coach Pete Carroll makes yoga and meditation sessions available to all players.

2014 Former Olympic track-and-field champion Carl Lewis embraces aerial yoga and incorporates it into the training program of the University of Houston track-and-field team.

2015 The UN General Assembly designates June 21 International Day of Yoga.

2016 NBA star Kobe Bryant says his decision to retire came through meditation, an integral part of yoga.

COMMON YOGA TERMS AND PHRASES

Every sport has its own language, and yoga is no different. Walking into your first class can feel like entering a foreign country. Since yoga originated in India, the names of the postures (or asanas) are in Sanskrit—not American's second language of choice. Some teachers will be kind enough to use English translations (as I do throughout this book), while others will assume you have mastered the basic Sanskrit terminology, such as *adho mukha svanasana*. (Say what? Oh, downward dog.) One of the fastest ways to tell whether you'll be able to connect with a teacher is to see how the teacher's language strikes you. I've had teachers use phrases like "widen your love canal" and "flower your buttocks," while other teachers have dropped the F-bomb and referred to my "big ass." Find a teacher you can relate to. That said, if you're stuck in a class where you have no idea what the teacher is talking about, you can always peek up to see what others in the class are doing, and if you still feel lost, just wave the teacher over and ask for help.

Asana. The literal meaning is "seat," but asana can refer to any pose or posture, such as plow pose or child's pose. "Moving through a series of asanas," refers to linking poses to the breath in a sequence like sun salutation A (page 88).

Bandha. The contracting of certain muscle groups near the perineum (*mulabandha*), transverse abdominals (*uddiyana bandha*), and throat (*jalandhara bandha*) during certain poses or breath work to increase the flow of energy and sensation moving through the nervous system.

Chakras. Energy centers throughout the body. These correlate to bundles of nerves in the body known by modern anatomy as "plexus," which are believed to be connected to emotional and mental states.

Dosha. Constitutional body types based on the five elements: earth, water, fire, space, and air. *Vata* is a *dosha* that reflects elements of space and air. *Pitta* reflects elements of fire and water. *Kapha* reflects elements of water and earth.

Drishti. A gazing point that helps you avoid distraction so you can focus or keep your balance in poses like tree (page 173).

Floss the shoulders. Open the shoulder joints, usually with the help of a strap.

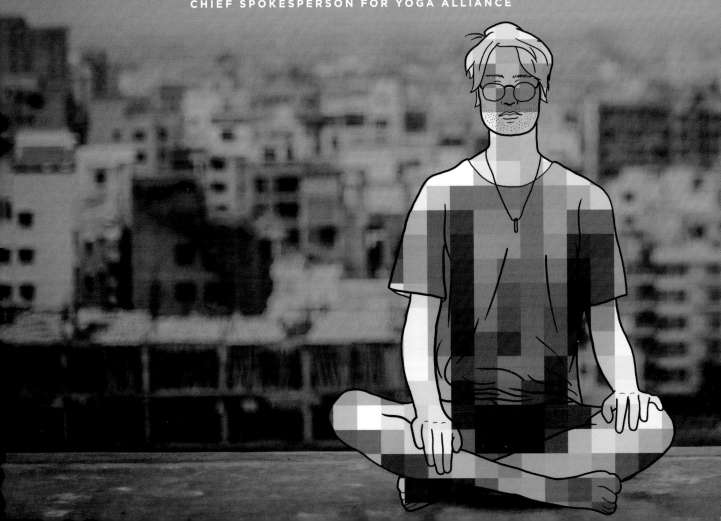

It is no coincidence that in the Yoga Sutras there are only 12 words about asana [posture] and they are very clear: 'Asana is steady and comfortable posture.' They don't say, Asana is contorting yourself into a pretzel for Instagram.

ANDREW TANNER

CHIEF SPOKESPERSON FOR YOGA ALLIANCE

Hug the midline. Draw into the core or center of the body to stabilize.

Kirtan. A form of devotional chanting.

Mantra. A sacred sound or phrase, like om.

Lion's breath. A breathing technique in which you open your mouth wide, stretch out your tongue, and exhale forcefully while making a distinct "ha" sound.

Melt your heart. Let go of tension in the chest area.

Mudra. A hand gesture used to direct the flow of energy in the body. *Gyan mudra*, done by connecting the thumb and forefinger tip to tip and relaxing the remaining fingers, is commonly used in seated position and is thought to improve concentration.

Namaste. A phrase that means "I bow to you," acknowledging the soul in one by the soul in another. Namaste is often spoken at the end of a yoga practice.

Om. Considered to be the first sound of creation; chanted at the beginning of the practice, the close, or both.

Pelvic floor. For men, the muscles that support the bladder and bowels.

Prana. Life force.

Pranayama. Breath work.

Root to rise. Press down into the foundation (for example, the feet or the sitting bones) to activate the muscles above it.

Sacrum. The small triangular bone at the base of the spine, directly above the tailbone.

Savasana. Also called corpse pose (page 132); often referred to as the most difficult pose because it involves simply lying in complete relaxation, with a quiet mind.

Shanti. The practice is often closed by chanting *shanti*, which means "peace."

Sitting bones Also called sit bones; the bony protrusions under the butt.

Soften the ribs. Drop the front of the rib cage toward the pelvis (in other words, stop arching the lower back and sticking out the butt).

Sternum. Also known as the breastbone; runs vertically down the center of the chest.

Sutra: An aphoristic statement summarizing a Vedic teaching.

Tapas. Self-discipline or purification through discipline or the heat generated by yogic practice; for some people, sitting still in meditation requires *tapas*.

Third eye. A reference to the chakra between the eyebrows.

Ujjayi. A hissing or "oceanic"-sounding breath, used to connect movement and quiet the mind.

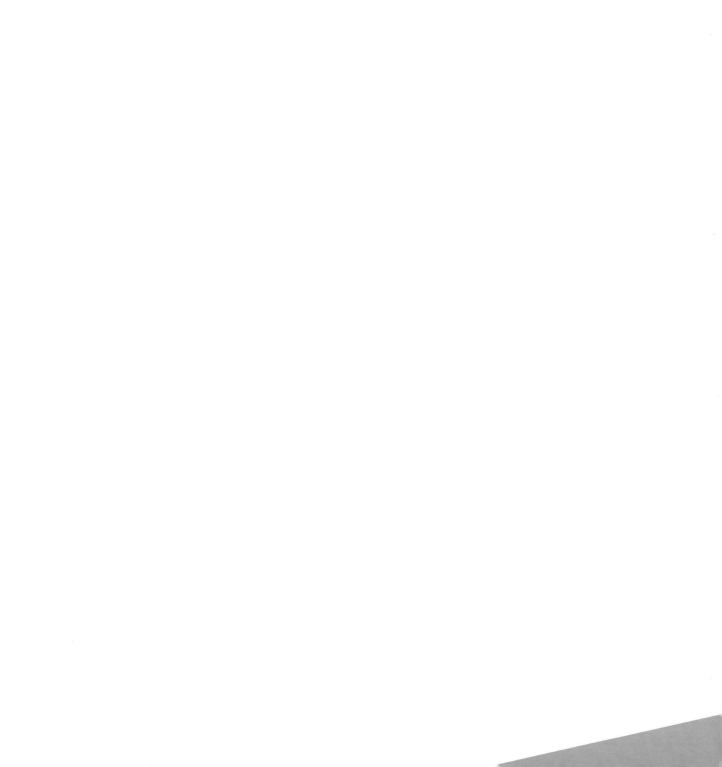

CHAPTER 2

WHY YOGA?

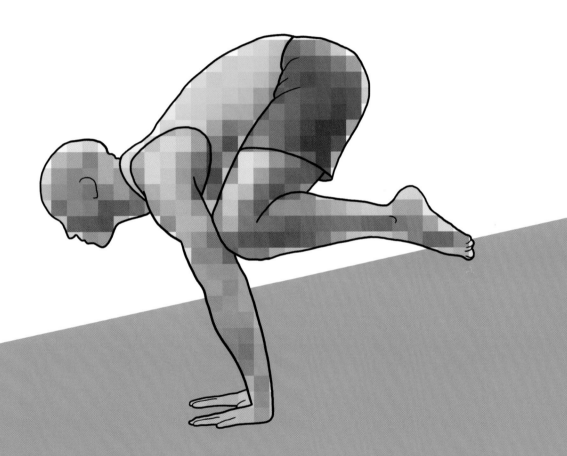

There are only twenty-four hours in a day, and in that stretch we're supposed to sleep at least eight hours, work at least another eight (but we all know it's more like ten to fourteen), do some form of cardiovascular exercise for at least thirty minutes, do some form of strength training, eat healthy meals, devote time to our loved ones, and, oh yeah, try to relax somewhere in between. And now I'm telling you to add yoga to the mix.

It's easy to look at your schedule and say, "There just isn't time." But there's always time when you prioritize. Yoga doesn't have to be a ninety-minutes-per-day, seven-days-a-week commitment. You'll still get benefits from even just ten minutes of yoga one day a week. If it helps, think of yoga as your opportunity to take a little vacation. It's time just for you, away from life's stresses. For as much time as you can spare, you get to turn off your cell phone, disconnect from the world, and focus only on you. It may sound indulgent—or even cheesy—but it's really just simple self-care.

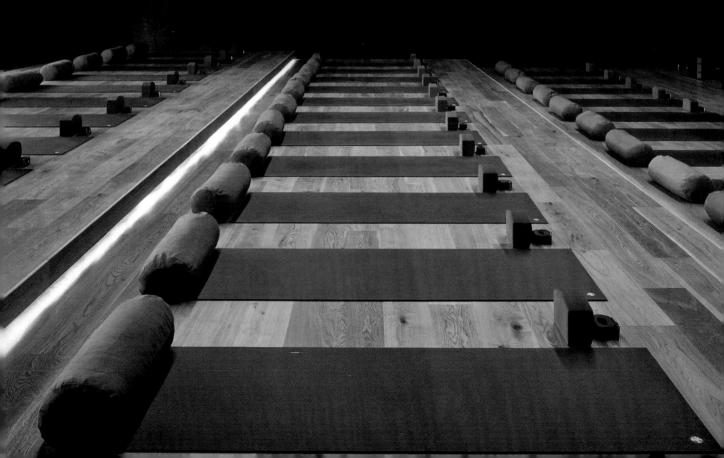

I actually really don't like doing yoga. You go stand in a 105-degree room and hold poses. It's not fun, like surfing. But I like how yoga makes me feel. I'm don't know if I've become more flexible, but I know I'm not getting stiffer.

TOM SERVAIS

SURF PHOTOGRAPHER

You may think you're strong, but yoga strength is different than gym strength. While many foundational yoga poses, such as plank and chair mimic strength exercises you might do at the gym, other poses, like half-moon or crow, help strengthen and develop areas we rarely work at the gym, like our wrists and our balance. Yoga is a great way to discover your body's imbalances. For example, do you wobble in warrior 3 on the right side but not the left? Do your hips sink when you hold side plank on the left side but not on the right? Once you become aware of these imbalances, you can start working toward achieving a more balanced body. We all know core strength is crucial for a healthy spine, and nothing engages the core like yoga. Just try holding boat pose for ten breaths. Learning how to engage your core and stabilizing muscles won't just help you master advanced poses like handstand, it will also help you move more efficiently and avoid injury.

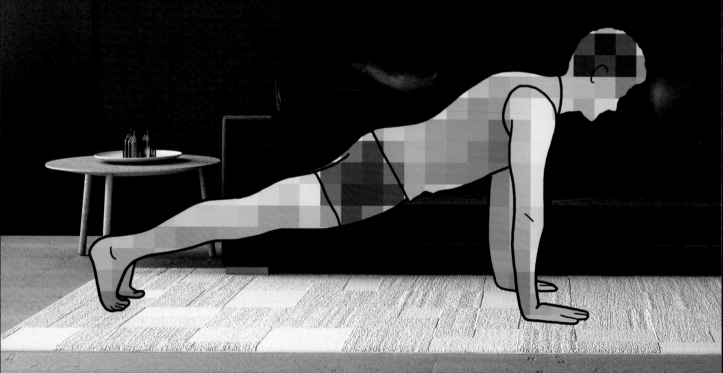

MICHAEL BEATRICE

HUSBAND, FATHER, AND LAPSED YOGI

When I started placekicking in college football, there was a high demand for me to achieve and maintain an extreme level of flexibility. My kicking power came from my ability to pull my leg back as far as possible, transfer the energy as quickly as possible through the ball, and follow through as far as possible with my leg. To withstand the stress of this whiplike motion and the impact on my plant leg, I'd stretch for a minimum of ninety minutes before a game. Some said that was crazy, but I can tell you I needed it. My power wasn't from an abundance of muscle; it was from this ability to harvest every ounce of my body's potential energy, and I always felt that stretching was the key. All that stretching led me to look for a source of strength building that could increase my flexibility. I turned to a free campus yoga class to explore strength and power and discovered I was a natural. However, while I could easily do arm balances, my core was never strong enough, even at my peak fitness, to hold a plank pose or elevate my body to achieve certain higher-level poses, but I always tried. I loved that yoga gave me another opportunity to try, show off, and "win."

When I started my career, I stopped going to yoga classes. I'm married, have a kid, and often work until 2 a.m. I prioritize work and family—and workouts that involve running or weight lifting. But any chance I get, I take the time to stretch, and usually those stretches are a yoga pose or two. Yoga is a holistic engagement of your body in a uniquely physical and mental way. Plus, it forces your mind to focus only on your body: what are you feeling at this exact moment? When I practiced regularly, I knew if the top of my left calf was tighter than normal or if my right hip flexor was a little loose and sliding out of place. People talk about oneness and the spiritual aspect of yoga. For me, it was never about that, but in a way I guess it was. My oneness was not with others or a higher power; it was with myself and my whole body. Know thyself, I guess. I regret that I fell out of the practice.

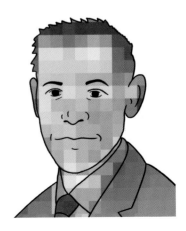

YOGA TO ADVANCE YOUR GAME

Whether you're a weekend warrior or a professional athlete, it's likely that your sport of choice beats up your body. Think of yoga as a complement to any sport. Yoga styles like Iyengar can heighten your awareness of muscle imbalances and areas of weakness. Vinyasa or Bikram can help strengthen your core and stabilizing muscles and also sharpen your focus. Learning to channel your breath on the mat will translate to smarter, more efficient breathing off the mat, whether you're a runner, cyclist, swimmer, or boxer. And restorative styles of yoga, such as yin, act like a delicious massage that targets connective tissues deep in the body.

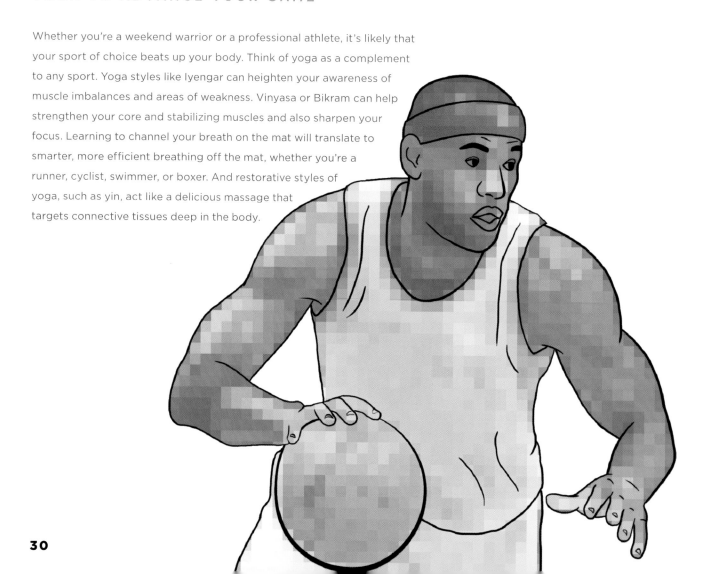

CHARLIE COYLE

FORWARD FOR THE NHL'S MINNESOTA WILD

The summer before I joined the Minnesota Wild, I attended a summer development camp. Our trainer mentioned that there was a yoga studio down the street and offered to set us up with classes. It wasn't mandatory, but I figured that there had to be some benefit. It was tough, hot power yoga. The amount of sweat that poured out of me was unbelievable. I felt so good after class. Me and some of the guys on the team started going twice a week. We'd skate, hit the weights, then go to yoga. I felt the best I'd ever felt on the ice that summer.

Finding my comfort zone in poses through my breathing helped me on the ice. I learned to slow my heart rate down before going back on the ice. In the weight room I can focus more on my breathing when I'm lifting because of yoga. The flexibility aspect of yoga is huge for hockey players. I don't know if humans are made to skate. Our hips are so tight. Pigeon pose has done wonders for my hips. The more you use your muscles, the tighter you get—all the more reason to do yoga.

DAVE KALAMA

WATERMAN AND BIG-WAVE SURFER

Like most guys in the late 1990s and early 2000s, my conceptual understanding of yoga was that it was soft, wussy stretching full of emotional yada yada. My first exposure to yoga was at a Quiksilver training camp that focused on the physical side of the practice. It kicked my butt. In fact, I pushed myself so hard that I hurt my back. That turned me off from the practice. But three years later, Laird Hamilton asked me to do yoga with him. He seemed committed, so I thought it was worth another try. This time the experience was much closer to what I expected yoga to be about—breathing, focus, balance— but the physical exertion in simple movements really blew me away. I was sweating so hard during that first session with Laird that when I left the studio I looked like I'd stepped out of a swimming pool. It wasn't even a heated class! Of course, I approached it like a typical young man with no yoga experience, muscling through every pose with no acknowledgment of my body's limits and trying to overcome every situation with bravado rather than breath. Breath instruction was foreign to me. To breathe during these very intense movements seemed impossible. I was so winded I had to huff and puff to get air in. It was a very humbling experience and completely changed my perception of yoga—and it got me hooked.

There's nothing wussy about yoga. It's very tough and very physical but leaves you feeling somewhere between euphoric and relaxed. I immediately noticed a difference in my paddling. In those days, there was this one guy who was just a bit faster than me. Eight times out of ten he'd beat me. But if I did yoga the morning before we raced, I would absolutely smoke him. That was the tipping point for me, and I started practicing yoga regularly. I'd never been that fast on a paddleboard. Yoga really translates to sports. With all of the water sports I do, whether surfing or paddling, I'm in a very fluid situation calculating data—speed, time, distance, and how I relate to a wave—at a subconscious level. When your subconscious is relaxed and free from stress or outside thoughts, you can make better decisions. Basically, you get in the flow more easily. The hardest part for me is finding time. But even if I do just fifteen minutes of yoga, it helps me so much.

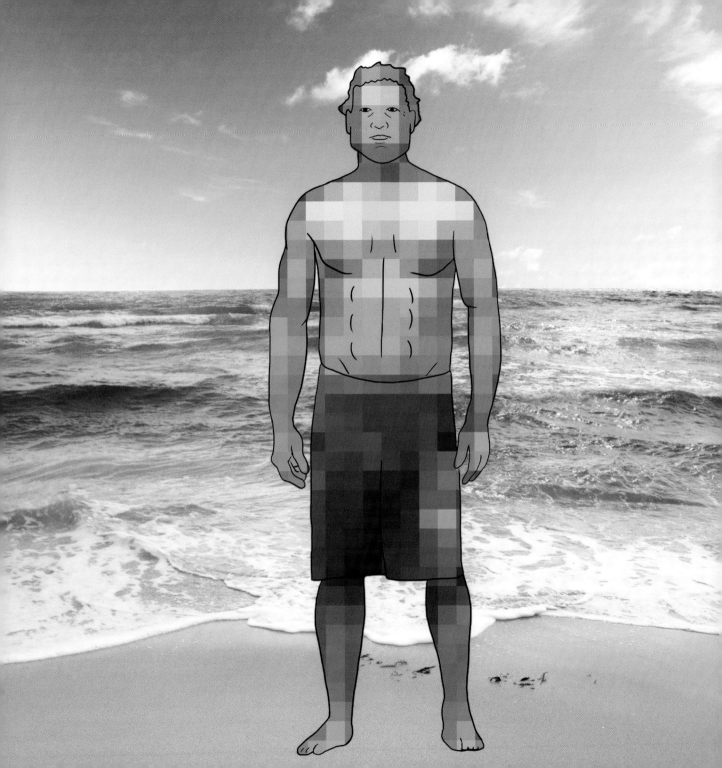

EXPERT ADVICE

(ON YOGA FOR RUNNERS)

Runners benefit from yoga in a number of ways. First, yoga stretches can often ease the pain associated with running. Oftentimes tight iliotibial (IT) bands can cause knee pain, which prevents runners from reaching their full potential. The same is true for sciatica, caused by a tight gluteus medius muscle or back pain that's the result of tension in the quadratus lumborum (QL). Second, yoga addresses poor posture, which can lead not only to discomfort but to shallow breathing. In addition, the breath work exercises help runners develop a kind of rhythmic breathing that can help reduce anxiety leading up to and during a race. Breath work can also facilitate better pacing throughout the race.

—KILEY HOLLIDAY
TEACHER OF YOGA FOR ATHLETES AND YOGA FOR RUNNERS

THREE POSES FOR RUNNERS

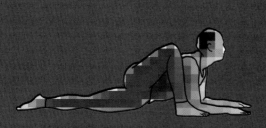
Lizard pose (page 152)

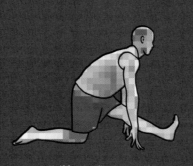
Half front splits (page 146)

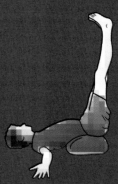
Legs up the wall (page 151)

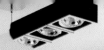

MYLES FENNON

MARATHONER AND ULTRARUNNER

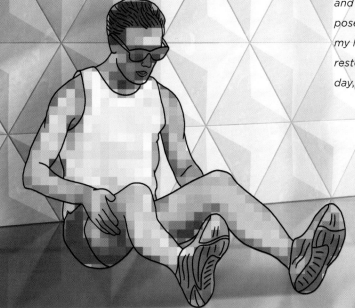

My real yoga breakthrough came when I signed up for a four-session yoga workshop for runners. I average fifty miles per week when I'm training for a one-hundred-miler, and figured I should do something that didn't beat up my body. Classes were elementary slow flows. We spent a lot of time in postures and moved slowly between them. My first impression was, "This is really hard for me." I didn't have the upper body strength for a lot of the poses, and I wasn't able to control my breath. But I liked how there was this crescendo to build yourself up to your edge and then slowly come back down. I also liked the routine of coming to a quiet place for an hour so I could relax and

hit the reset button. The running-specific classes made regular classes less intimidating for me, and I started going to a more intense, heated vinyasa class. It was fucking hard. I looked like such a rookie next to these girls effortlessly flinging their bodies around. That's when I really started to appreciate the breathing aspect of yoga. I knew my body had reached its limit when my breath broke down. The quality of my breath was a signal to ease back or try a different variation, and I've learned to channel that when I run. I haven't gotten injured in years, and I think yoga has a lot to do with that. It counterbalances the tightening that running creates in my muscles, and it's taught me more innovative ways to stretch. Lizard pose helps my tight hips, standing forward fold stretches my lower back and hamstrings, and legs up the wall is restorative for my legs. I try to do these three poses every day, even if it's at home while watching TV.

EXPERT ADVICE

(ON YOGA FOR CYCLISTS)

The trash talking that happens on the bike quickly comes to an end when I get guys on the mat. They head straight to the back row because they are so tight and hate not being good at something. Cyclists tend to have tight hamstrings, hips, and shoulders and a tight lower back. When you're on a bike, your body is in an unnatural state. You're hunched over, rounding the back and dropping the shoulders. Your hips are in flexion, and your hamstrings and glutes are getting worked hard. Yoga helps open the body up after it's been crunched forward for so long. It undoes all of the damage from the bike. It also builds strength, particularly in stabilizing muscles like the hips, groins, and ankles. Most cyclists take up yoga for the flexibility, but once they start practicing they find that the breath work and focus translate back to the bike. Maintaining rhythmic breathing on a climb or during a sprint requires endurance and keeping calm under pressure. Yoga trains just that.

—MADONNA BLASUCCI
YOGA INSTRUCTOR AT GEORGE HINCAPIE'S DOMESTIQUE CYCLING CAMPS

THREE POSES FOR CYCLISTS

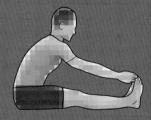

Seated forward fold (page 164)

Pigeon pose (page 155)

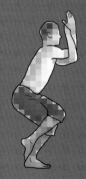

Eagle pose (page 139)

SEAMUS MULLEN

CHEF AND AVID MOUNTAIN BIKER

I tried practicing vinyasa yoga when I was suffering from rheumatoid arthritis and ended up feeling worse. I was too stiff and tight from the inflammation in my body. So I tried restorative yoga and it helped my body calm down. I was able to relax slowly into poses with the aid of blocks and bolsters. As I progressed, I got interested in learning more about the practice. Now I do flows on my own every day. I feel it helps me in other physical aspects of my life. It's improved my running and cycling. Understanding the breath is huge. We're not really taught that in sports. I use ujjayi *breath when I'm climbing hills on my bike. It helps me control my oxygen intake, and I think that has a direct correlation to clearing lactic acid and recovering more quickly. In cycling, you're in this hunched position that restricts your breathing, and when you get into uncomfortable situations, like a big climb, you tighten up. Whether you're on a bike, in the kitchen, in the dentist's chair, or about to get a tattoo, your whole body tenses when you're faced with stress. Everything is clenched and you need to remind yourself to breathe.*

I've tried to apply what I learn from yoga to my daily life. It's helped me a lot during my bike commute in New York City, where basically everyone is trying to kill you. There is real value in learning to channel your emotion through breathing and to let others' anger swim past you. Through visualization, I've learned

to lead with the breath and consider movement before making a movement. This helps me in handstand. I see myself in the position before I move into it. When I'm on my bike and someone clips me, I could easily reply with anger, fire, and fury, but instead I just breathe.

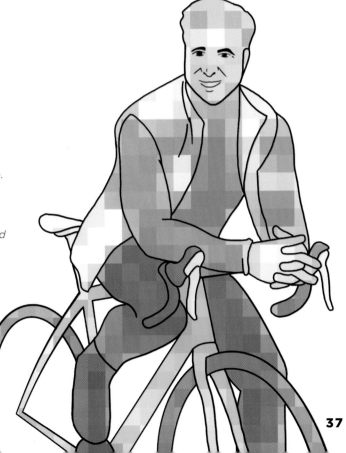

THE MIND-BODY CONNECTION

The majority of people come to yoga in search of the physical benefits. Perhaps their vanity is drawn to the toned triceps, tight abs, and effortless handstands they see pictured on the cover of *Yoga Journal*. Without a doubt, yoga will increase your flexibility, muscle strength, and athletic performance. But once you start practicing, you'll see benefits that extend far beyond the physical.

Unlike stretching or many types of exercise, yoga isn't just about physical movement or postures. Yoga is unique because it connects the mind and body to the rhythm of the breath, which in turn helps us direct our attention inward to become more self-aware. And in our fast-paced, high-stress, digitally enhanced world, it's more important than ever to slow down and examine how we're feeling, both physically and mentally. Yoga helps us recognize habitual patterns: Do we tighten our shoulders when we're in uncomfortable situations? Do we push ourselves too far, or can we accept our limitations?

Whether you're a professional athlete, weekend warrior, or well-intentioned couch potato, yoga will help you pick up on your personal strengths, weaknesses, and imbalances. The practice trains you to tune in to the subtleties of your body.

At a deeper level, the mindfulness instilled through yoga, perhaps while trying to balance in half-moon or breathe fully in bow pose, has implications beyond the mat. Research suggests that meditation sharpens skills like attention and memory, cultivates emotional intelligence, and strengthens our ability to regulate our emotions (and therefore manage stress). It also enhances creativity, with studies suggesting that we come up with some of our biggest breakthroughs when in a relaxed state of mind. After a few yoga classes, you'll go from running a to-do list through your head to sitting up from *savasana* with a "eureka" moment. Look at some of the most successful men of our time: Steve Jobs, Steph Curry, Tom Brady, Tony Schwartz, Phil Jackson, Ray Dalio. What do they all have in common? They've made meditation part of their daily lives.

NATE DENISON

YOGA TEACHER

When I was a teenager, my hamstrings were so tight that it hindered my ability to play baseball, basketball, and soccer. I was really passionate about sports and had tried lots of things to loosen up, and then my mom suggested yoga. I was competitive, so I didn't like that I couldn't do a lot of the poses and ended up going back to stretching. After college I moved to New York City and started dating a girl who was really into yoga. She managed a really nice studio, Pure Yoga, and I got to take free classes. The relationship didn't work out, but I grew my practice from there and embraced Bikram. Even if I didn't know what I was doing with my career, my living situation, or my relationship, I could make it to class and practice. Thoughts would come up and I could let go of them, and when class was over, I could leave all of my worries on the mat and walk out the door with a little peace of mind. I might not have all of the answers to my life figured out, but I have a better sense of direction and self-awareness. There is something very powerful about being able to access that. Yoga doesn't just give you physical flexibility; it gives you mental flexibility. You become open to other ways of thinking or doing things. Now I teach yoga. I still can't do all of the postures, but I've realized that's not what makes a good teacher.

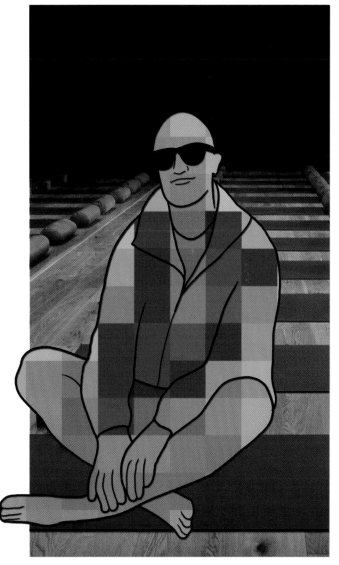

ARE YOGA AND MEDITATION THE SAME THING?

Most people hear the word "meditation" and picture a cross-legged Buddha with a beatific smile. However, meditation in its simplest form is really just mindfulness—and in the West, most of us could benefit from bringing more calm and focus into our crazy days. The Yoga Sutras state that yoga happens when the mind becomes quiet. This mental stillness is created by bringing the body, mind, and senses into balance, which relaxes the nervous system.

As traditional Eastern yoga has morphed into a more physical style in the West, meditation has taken a backseat. However, it's now becoming clear that stillness is as important to our health as movement is. Research has shown that people's minds tend to wander about 50 percent of the time. And as we become ever more enmeshed with email, text messages, social media, and other digital distractions, this will only increase the challenge of staying focused. Meditation training can help curb our tendency to get distracted.

You may wonder how, exactly, to go about meditating. Like yoga, meditation is a very personal practice, and there are many styles; there's really no right or wrong way to meditate. The main thing is to find time to relax your mind. Meditation is often incorporated into Western-style yoga classes, usually at the beginning or end of class. You'll know when you've figured it out because you'll feel a deep sense of calm and a renewed mind upon finishing, sort of like coming back from a two-week vacation.

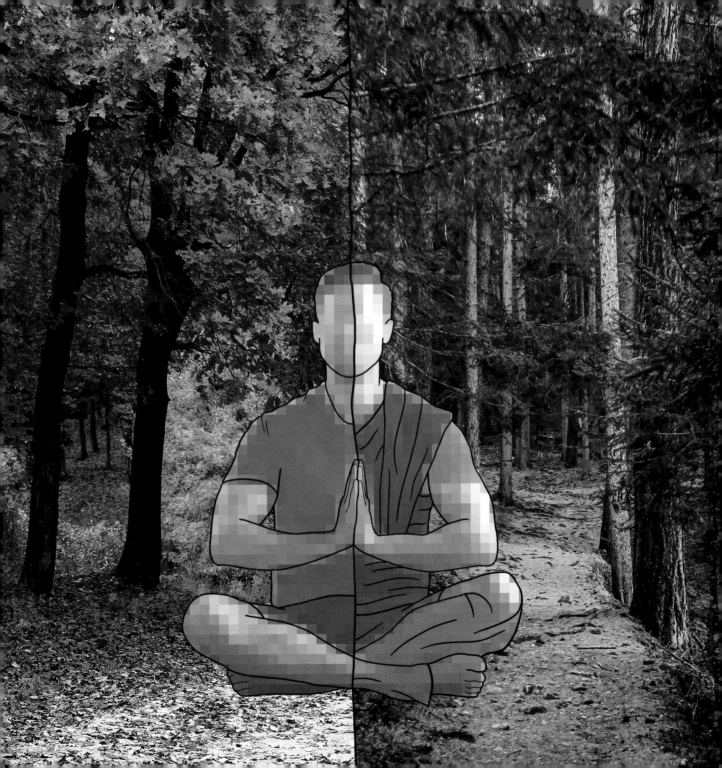

EXPERT ADVICE

(ON MEDITATION)

People think meditation is not thinking or making the mind go blank. That's not true. You cannot not think. Even highly practiced meditators have thoughts when they meditate. Sometimes there are moments without thought, but this isn't the goal of meditation. The purpose is to notice what's happening within you, to be in the present moment even for just a minute or two, and simply reflect. This is time to ask big questions: 'Who am I?' 'What is my purpose?' 'What makes me happy?' There are many ways to reach this place within. Breathing, calm music, and guided meditation can reduce stress by 50 percent or more. I always say breathing is the gateway to meditation.

—DORON LIBSHTEIN
FOUNDER OF THE MENTORS CHANNEL, A WEBSITE FOR PERSONAL GROWTH

DORON LIBSHTEIN'S TIPS ON HOW TO START MEDITATING

Set aside time daily. For beginners, start by setting aside fifteen to twenty minutes each day. It's best to meditate in the morning or just before you go to bed at night. You may want to split your time and do seven to ten minutes both in the morning and at night. The timing isn't as important as just doing it regularly.

Use a mantra. A mantra (like "om," "om shanti om," or "I am peace") can give you something to focus on during meditation. Just repeat your mantra, whatever it is, on the inhalation and the exhalation. But if you don't feel like using a mantra, it's not a requirement.

Follow your breath. Your breath is another tool that can help you focus, and it's also important for stress reduction. For example, lengthening the exhalation promotes a state of calm. Try using four counts on each inhalation and eight counts on each exhalation. However, your breath shouldn't be strained in any way, so if you need to work up to eight counts, that's fine. Be aware that it's normal for the mind to wander away from the breath at times. When that happens, just bring your attention gently back to the breath.

Try guided meditation. Many people do better when someone guides them on their meditation journey, whether at a studio, like Inscape in New York City, or via an app like Headspace or a podcast like Meditation Oasis.

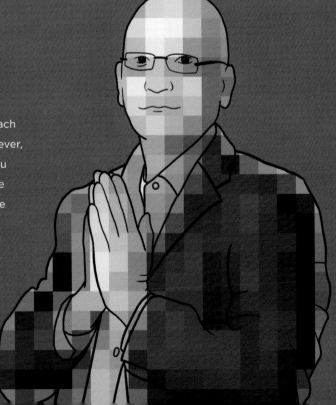

YOGA AS THERAPY

Yoga can deliver much more than increased flexibility and a stronger core. In many ways yoga is both medication and preventative care. Somewhere between 75 and 90 percent of all visits to the doctor are for stress-related ailments. But why pay for meds—and risk the side effects—when you may be able to stave off stress with yoga? The simple act of lowering your head below your heart in a pose like standing forward fold calms the brain, which helps relieve stress. Studies have linked meditation to reduced dependency on opioid drugs and decreased depression. Research has also shown that yoga reduces risk factors for chronic diseases such as heart disease and high blood pressure, and that it alleviates chronic conditions such as insomnia, back pain, and anxiety. In the long run, the time you put into yoga will pay you back with more time (and save you money).

The medical field has started to embrace yoga as an alternative therapy for people suffering from post-traumatic stress symptoms, addiction, and traumatic brain injury. A study conducted by Harvard Medical School and funded by the U.S. Department of Defense found that veterans diagnosed with post-traumatic stress disorder showed improvement in their symptoms after ten weeks of yoga classes, done twice a week, and fifteen minutes of daily practice at home. Studies conducted by Roy King, an associate professor of psychiatry and behavioral science at Stanford University, have shown a correlation between yoga and inhibition of the dopamine surge addicts experience from using drugs. King has also found that deep breathing patterns in certain forms of yoga, such as Kundalini, have the power to release the body's natural pleasure-producing endorphins, acting as a substitute for a drug-induced high.

The more I practiced yoga, the more my various unhealthy coping mechanisms like drugs and alcohol eventually gave way to healthier alternatives that didn't hinge on self-abuse. Long, late nights were replaced by early mornings, mind numbing by mind opening. Once I surrendered to the beautiful riptide of yoga and all of its component pieces, I never wanted to return to chaos.

CHAD DENNIS

DIRECTOR OF YOGA FOR WANDERLUST HOLLYWOOD

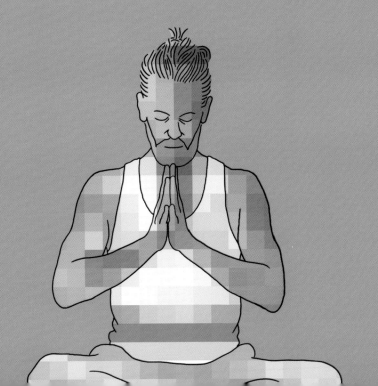

YOGA FOR HEALING

After suffering a career-ending traumatic brain injury during a snowboard crash, Kevin Pearce, a former professional snowboarder, embraced yoga as part of his recovery. He also cofounded the LoveYourBrain Foundation, a nonprofit organization that helps improve the quality of life of people affected by brain injury. Subsequently, LoveYourBrain partnered with Dartmouth University to conduct a pilot study to determine which aspects of yoga most benefit people with traumatic brain injuries. LoveYourBrain Yoga, a gentle style that integrates guided meditation, breathing exercises, and physical postures, was developed based on the study's findings. In 2016, this new style of adaptive yoga started being offered in studios throughout the United States.

KEVIN PEARCE

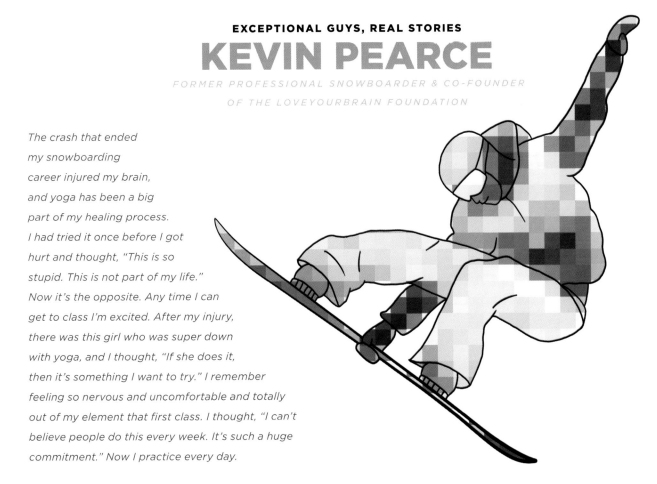

The crash that ended my snowboarding career injured my brain, and yoga has been a big part of my healing process. I had tried it once before I got hurt and thought, "This is so stupid. This is not part of my life." Now it's the opposite. Any time I can get to class I'm excited. After my injury, there was this girl who was super down with yoga, and I thought, "If she does it, then it's something I want to try." I remember feeling so nervous and uncomfortable and totally out of my element that first class. I thought, "I can't believe people do this every week. It's such a huge commitment." Now I practice every day.

My injury left me with double vision. Yoga has really helped to improve that. We all hear about how yoga connects the mind and body. That connection heals. In life, we're always being judged. With my brain injury, so many things can go wrong in daily life. The yoga studio is a totally safe place where no one is critical of you. Maybe you don't make it all the way into the pose or hold the pose for five counts. It doesn't matter. When I first started, I was really stoked on hot, power vinyasa classes.

But the longer I practice, the more I've realized that I'm not doing yoga to get superstrong or to get a workout. I'm going to chill and relax and focus on my breath. Now I really love yin and restorative classes. The teachers aren't trying to get you into handstand or intense postures. They try to get you to be intensely relaxed. I've learned that we can't stop thinking, but we can slow down our thinking, and that relaxes the brain. When I go to slow flow or yin class, I find this trancelike state that's really peaceful.

YOGA FOR DETOX

Yoga can help make amends for a binge of booze or greasy food. When you twist your body, you're compressing your abdominal organs, including all of your digestive organs. Think of it as wringing out all of the toxins. This pressure helps push toxins from the kidneys, liver, and spleen and move stagnant blood. Then, when you come out of the twist, these organs get a new supply of oxygen-rich blood, which stimulates digestion and metabolism. Yoga won't cure your hangover, but it can act like a cleanse so you don't have to suffer through a liquid diet of juice. Try to remember to twist from the right to left to mimic the flow of digestion.

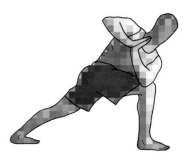

Revolved crescent lunge (page 162)

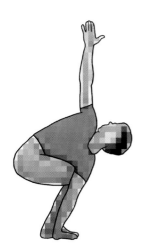

Revolved chair (page 161)

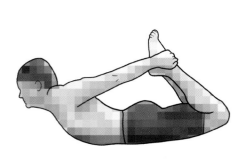

Bow pose (page 123)

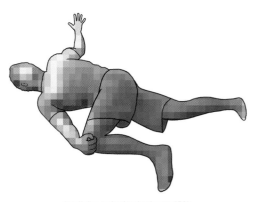

Reclining spinal twist (page 159)

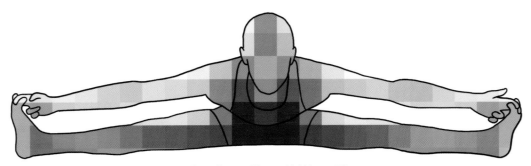

Wide-angle seated forward fold (page 179)

CHAPTER 3

WHICH YOGA?

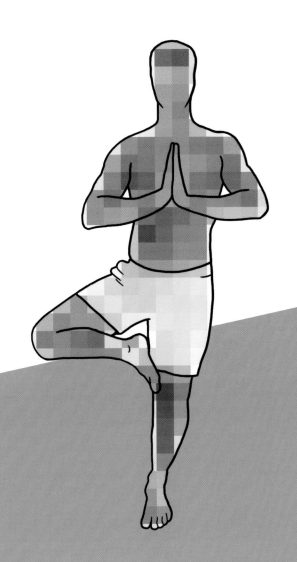

FIND YOUR YOGA STYLE

The explosion of dozens of new yoga styles in recent years has made yoga—a practice meant to alleviate stress—more stressful, particularly for beginners. Don't get overwhelmed. The variety of options out there means there's a style that's ideal for you. However, just as with dating, it might take a few tries before you find a great match.

Luckily, there are some filters that can help you weed out the mismatches ahead of time. Start by asking yourself what you want to get out of the practice. Are you looking for a sweaty, invigorating, strength-building practice? Or do you want a more restorative, therapeutic, meditative practice? Does the thought of chanting and hugging your neighbor make you want to run out of the room, or do you want to embrace a more spiritual, communal practice? Think of the information in this chapter as your cheat sheet for the core styles of yoga. Once you settle on one you like, try offshoots, and remember that you don't need to be faithful to one style. You may find that a combination of styles works best for you.

Asking someone what style of yoga they do is an invalid question.
You either do yoga or you don't.

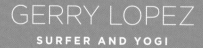

GERRY LOPEZ
SURFER AND YOGI

GERRY LOPEZ

SURFER AND YOGI

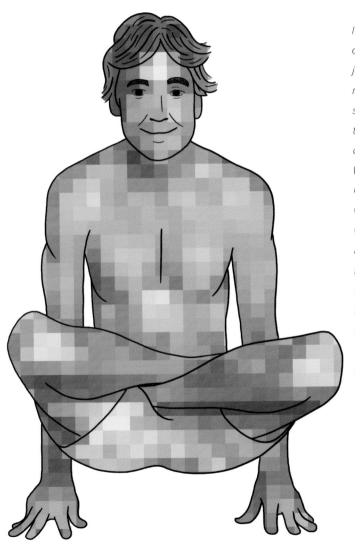

In the 1960s I was a hippie surfer attending the University of Hawaii. I went to a yoga class and knew immediately, just by watching the teacher move, that it would help my surfing. I thought that if I could move like that on a surfboard, I could really shift with the wave. Back then there weren't many yoga studios; you were pretty much on your own. So I bought and studied The Complete Illustrated Book of Yoga, *by Swami Vishnu-devananda. Over the decades I've developed a personal practice, which I do first thing every morning, even though that's when my body is stiffest. Surfing is all about flexibility and core strength. Lying down and paddling on the board isn't conducive to correct breathing, so having a* pranayama *practice has really helped me improve my breathing while paddling. I like big waves, and being able to be calm and hold my breath in wipeout situations has been very beneficial. Yoga hasn't just improved my surfing; it's improved my life. Being aware, centered, and present is where we all should be. Unfortunately, most of us are not. Everybody needs yoga, but not everyone understands that.*

POPULAR YOGA STYLES, DEFINED

Acro-yoga. This is a blend of yoga, acrobatics, dance, Thai massage, and body-weight strength training. It's a partner-based practice that builds not just strength and flexibility, but also trust. If you've ever propped your kid up on your feet to play Superman, you've done acro-yoga.

> **Best for:** Couples; ex-gymnasts; guys who want to build strength; guys who get bored easily; guys with hip or back pain
>
> **Devotee:** Tim Ferriss, best-selling author and entrepreneur

Aerial. Also called antigravity yoga, aerial yoga combines acrobatics with traditional yoga postures performed in the air with the support of soft, hammock-like silks. Because hanging upside down helps decompress the spine, it promotes finding more length in the spine. It also allows for more ease in inversions and better alignment in challenging postures.

> **Best for:** Guys with Cirque du Soleil fantasies; guys with back pain; guys who want a restorative practice
>
> **Devotee:** Carl Lewis, track-and-field superstar

Ashtanga. This athletic, vigorous practice consists of a series of poses performed in specific sequences synchronized to the breath. Be warned: It helps to have an understanding of fundamental postures before jumping into an ashtanga class; try a private class first, or start with slower, alignment-focused classes to wrap your head around the basics.

> **Best for:** Fit type A guys looking for a challenge; athletes
>
> **Devotees:** Alex Martins, Brazilian big-wave surfer; Terje Håkonsen, Norwegian professional snowboarder; the Texas Rangers baseball team

Bikram. Akin to doing yoga in a sauna, Bikram is sweaty and stinky. Each ninety-minute class consists of a series of twenty-six postures, done in a systematic order, in a room heated to 104 degrees. The heat may make you feel like Gumby, so be careful not to overstretch and injure yourself.

> **Best for:** Fit type A and OCD personalities; guys who thinks sweat is a requirement of a workout; athletes; guys in need of a detox
>
> **Devotees:** Garrett McNamara, big-wave surfer; David Beckham, soccer superstar; Kareem Abdul-Jabbar, nineteen-time NBA All-Star

Forrest Yoga. This hot practice combines physically challenging sequences with deep emotional exploration. Founder Ana Forrest developed poses and sequences that address emotional pain, as well as physical ailments that result from our modern lifestyle, such as carpal tunnel syndrome, intestinal disorders, and chronic back and shoulder pain. Classes focus on building core strength and internal heat.

> **Best for:** Guys looking for the emotional benefits of yoga combined with a more physical practice; guys who struggle with abuse or addiction; guys suffering from chronic physical pain caused by lifestyle; guys looking for personal transformation
>
> **Devotees:** The Exalted Warrior Foundation, a nonprofit that facilitates adaptive yoga programs for wounded warriors in military and veterans hospitals

Hatha. Traditionally, "hatha" was the umbrella term for any physical yoga practice. Today, it often refers to a style of class focused on breath work, proper alignment, and calming the mind. Ashtanga, Iyengar, vinyasa, and power yoga are all types of hatha yoga.

> **Best for:** Beginners looking to master basic breathing techniques and poses; guys worried that they aren't flexible enough for yoga; stressed-out dads or executives
>
> **Devotees:** Ryan Giggs, former Manchester United soccer star

Iyengar. This alignment-focused style of yoga uses props to help students achieve correct alignment. Don't be surprised if you only do a handful of poses during a sixty-minute class. The emphasis is on learning the subtle movements that can help you go deeper into a pose and gaining greater physical awareness.

> **Best for:** Yoga purists; perfectionists; guys working with injuries or structural imbalances; beginners looking for a sound foundation of fundamentals before advancing to faster-paced styles; guys looking for a more restorative class
>
> **Devotees:** Germany's World Cup–winning 2014 soccer team

Jivamukti. The name Jivamukti is an adaptation of the Sanskrit word *jivanmukti*, which means "liberation while living." In this approach to yoga, founded in 1985 by David Life and Sharon Gannon, teachers encourage students to apply yogic philosophies like *ahimsa*, or nonharming, to their daily lives. The athletic, vinyasa-inspired practice focuses on spiritual development. Be prepared to embrace chanting, references to spiritual texts, meditation, and discussions on how veganism leads to joy.

> **Best for:** Activists; vegans; guys who are drawn to the spiritual side of yoga but want a more athletic practice
>
> **Devotee:** Russell Simmons, pioneering hip-hop producer

STEVEN NYMAN

PROFESSIONAL SKIER

I've always been attracted to a holistic approach to training. I started practicing yoga when I was in my twenties and noticed I skied better, so I integrated it into my program. In recent years our team's trainer has focused on more than just fine-tuning our physical strength. For example, he'll have us do a fast circuit, then stand on a slackline to train our bodies to balance under fatigue. I realized that this is kind of what yoga is doing. By the end of a class, you're fatigued but really focusing to stay balanced. That's probably why I've benefited so much over the years from the practice. I think most guys do fast, hot yoga, but I prefer the classic, longer, slower yoga where you hold the poses. It helps with my focus, and I'll hold poses until I'm shaking. I go to a class in Park City where it's me and twenty women, but I don't care. It's what my body needs.

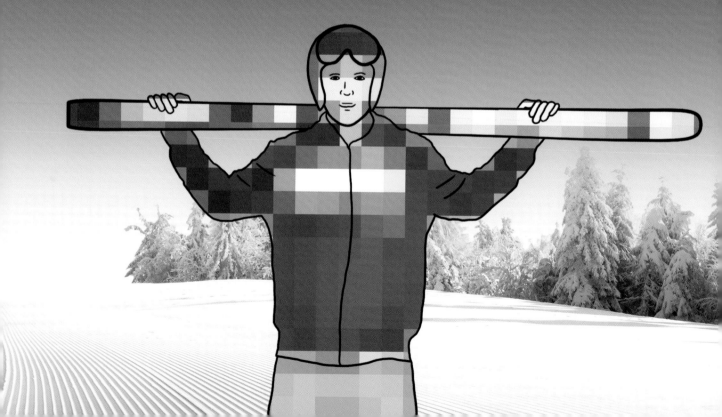

Kundalini. Also called the yoga of awareness, Kundalini is a blend of spiritual and physical practices developed to awaken the energy in the spine and help us achieve spiritual elevation and personal transformation. Classes incorporate chanting, singing, breathing exercises, *mudras*, and energetic movement-based postures. Don't be alarmed if everyone in class is dressed in white: founder Yogi Bhajan believed wearing white expanded a person's "auric radiance."

> **Best for:** Open-minded yogis looking to explore the spiritual side of the practice; guys interested in developing their breathing techniques; fans of white clothing
>
> **Devotees:** Russell Brand, British actor and iconoclast; Khajak Keledjian, cofounder of the luxury fashion retailer Intermix; Eddie George, former NFL player

Mysore. In Mysore yoga, a subset of ashtanga yoga, students can show up at any time during a three-hour window to do their own practice. Students flow at their own pace and to their own breath as a teacher moves around the room to offer personal adjustments.

> **Best for:** Fit type A guys; independent personalities; experienced ashtanga yogis who are already familiar with proper alignment and sequencing; guys looking for a more personalized approach to a vigorous practice
>
> **Devotees:** Daniel Loeb, hedge fund manager and founder of Third Point LLC

Power. Walt Baptiste, the founder of power yoga, believed that a physically challenging practice created a foundation for facing emotional challenges in life. Be prepared for a workout. Fast-paced flows will have your arms shaking and your heart rate rising. Classes are often performed in a heated room.

> **Best for:** Athletes; CrossFit junkies; guys looking to develop strength; guys looking to develop calm under pressure
>
> **Devotees:** The Philadelphia Eagles; the Hendrick Motorsports NASCAR racing team; David Carrier Porcheron, Canadian professional snowboarder

Tantric. When you hear the word "tantric," your mind may jump straight to sex, perhaps because this ancient practice has been linked to extended orgasms. While it may improve your sex life (believe it or not, spooning is a tantric position), the purpose of tantric yoga is actually to work on self-improvement through a powerful combination of mantras, postures, *mudras*, and energy work. The thinking here is that once you're in tune with who you are, you can deepen your relationship with your partner.

> **Best for:** Guys struggling with relationship issues; guys who want to bring yoga into the bedroom; anyone looking for a spiritual, transformational practice
>
> **Devotees:** Sting, one of the best-selling music artists of all time

Viniyoga. A therapeutic style of yoga tailored to individual needs, viniyoga is focused on mobilizing the spine and coordinating movement with the breath. Viniyoga emphasizes function over form and adapts postures to achieve desired results. The goal isn't to cure ailments, but to reduce and manage symptoms that cause suffering and to change attitudes that inhibit natural healing.

> **Best for:** Guys suffering from chronic pain; anyone looking for personal transformation; beginners looking to understand the basics; guys who want to develop a personal practice
>
> **Devotees:** Mark Bertolini, CEO of health insurance giant Aetna

Vinyasa. Often called vinyasa flow, this is a fast-paced practice where the breath is synchronized to a continuous flow of postures. Vinyasa has a dance-like quality and builds both strength and flexibility. Sequences are often choreographed to music.

> **Best for:** Athletes; guys looking for a challenging physical practice; guys looking to build strength and flexibility
>
> **Devotees:** Adam Levine, lead singer for Maroon 5

Yin. Jokingly called "sleepy time" yoga, yin yoga is all about relaxation. This form of restorative yoga emphasizes flexibility. Seated, passive postures target connective tissue around the joints, especially in the pelvis, hips, and lower spine. Postures can be held for as long as ten minutes each. Props are often used to initiate a deeper release while in postures. This is a great style for honing a meditation practice.

> **Best for:** Athletes looking to complement high-impact training; athletes rehabbing injuries; anyone looking to relieve tension in overworked joints; workaholics who need stress relief
>
> **Devotees:** Mike Adams, NFL safety with the Indianapolis Colts; Brian Detrick, professional water-skier

I had tried yoga once or twice, but the classes were too advanced and I never really got into the practice. Then I found myself going through a breakup and looking for something meditative. I saw a yoga DVD, and perhaps because I was a bit banged up emotionally, I was like, "Meditation, ritual, exercise—and cute girls!" It was a great way to learn the basics and maybe a way for me to safely connect with women on a daily basis. Early on I liked slow vinyasa. I exercise plenty, so I didn't need an intense workout, and it felt good to stretch my hypertight body, something I hadn't done after a workout since college. Yoga became a way for me to stay centered in the present moment, kind of like climbing, except yoga healed my body from the beating it took on the climbing wall or crag. Most forms of exercise break down the body but yoga is therapeutic. When my back had spasms a few years ago, I'm convinced that my simple, daily, restorative yoga practice was the true long-term and curative solution—more so than heat and muscle relaxers. I think a lot of guys who do yoga focus on how it can intensify their workouts. We forget how much we can benefit from opening up our bodies.

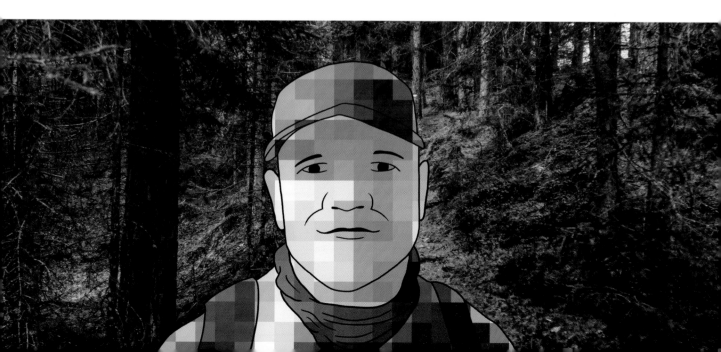

WHAT STYLE OF YOGA IS RIGHT FOR YOU?

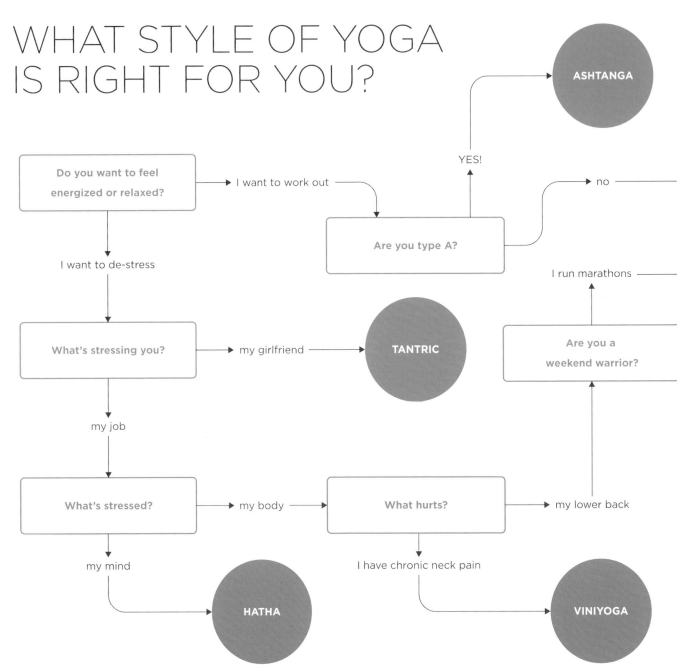

Do you want to feel energized or relaxed? → I want to work out → **Are you type A?**

Are you type A? → YES! → **ASHTANGA**

Are you type A? → no

Do you want to feel energized or relaxed? ↓ I want to de-stress

What's stressing you? → my girlfriend → **TANTRIC**

What's stressing you? ↓ my job

What's stressed? → my body → **What hurts?**

What hurts? → my lower back

What hurts? ↓ I have chronic neck pain → **VINIYOGA**

What's stressed? ↓ my mind → **HATHA**

Are you a weekend warrior? ↑ I run marathons

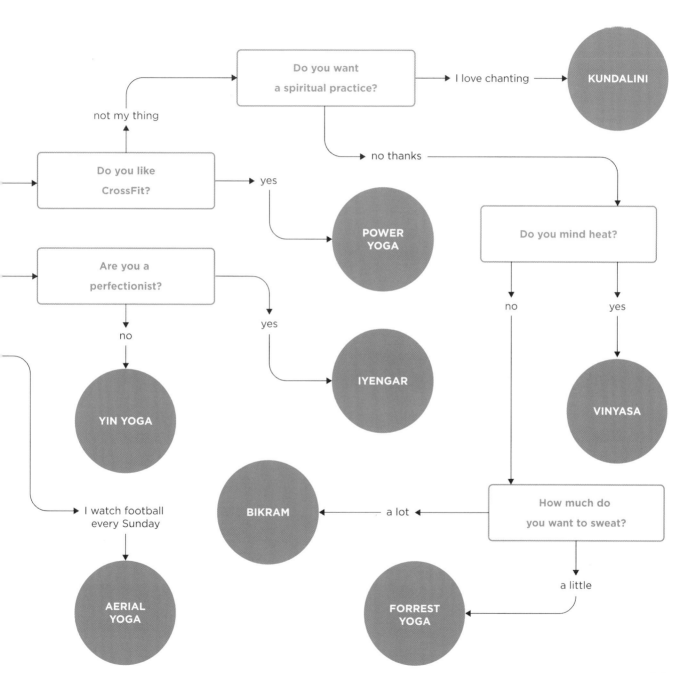

Do you want a spiritual practice? → I love chanting → **KUNDALINI**

not my thing

Do you like CrossFit? → yes

no thanks

Do you mind heat?

Are you a perfectionist?

POWER YOGA

no   yes

no

yes

IYENGAR

YIN YOGA

VINYASA

I watch football every Sunday

BIKRAM ← a lot ←

How much do you want to sweat?

a little

AERIAL YOGA

FORREST YOGA

61

CHAPTER 4

HOW YOGA?

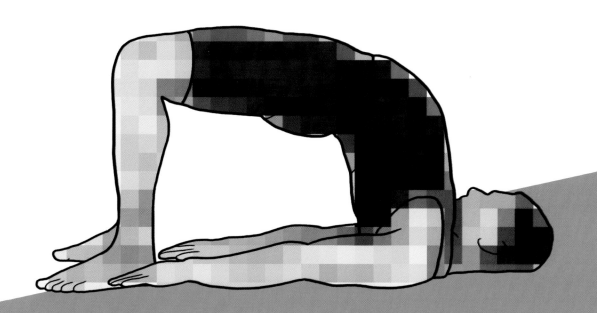

YOUR YOGA IS ONLY AS GOOD AS YOUR TEACHER

We've all had coaches we've loved and coaches we've loathed. Some motivate us; others make us feel like shit. Yoga teachers can be the same. Once you find a style of yoga that resonates with you, seek out a teacher you connect with. Each teacher has a unique focus, often inspired by where and with whom he or she has trained. A good teacher will make you feel comfortable in class, helping you focus on what you can do, rather than what you can't. It's one thing to correct someone in a pose; it's another to call a student out in front of the entire class for not being able to touch his or her head to the floor. A good teacher will also inquire about injuries before starting a class and will always ask permission before adjusting students. Sometimes the subtlest of adjustments or a new cue to enter a pose can help you achieve comfort in poses you once found agonizing.

Some instructors will speak in sports analogies, while others will reference spiritual texts. Find a teacher who speaks your language. I once had a teacher tell me that he'd spent nearly two hours tapping a bottle of wine against a wall during a retreat in Morocco so that pressure would build and the cork would pop out. When he described the task as focused meditation, I knew we'd get along. If you're looking to practice outside of a studio, look for a private teacher who's registered with the Yoga Alliance, or try DVDs from top-notch yoga teachers, like Rodney Yee or Eoin Finn.

TUNE IN TO THESE YOUTUBE YOGA CHANNELS

Whether you practice at home, on the road, or in a studio, these yoga channels offer guidance for both beginners and experienced yogis and will keep your practice fresh with different sequences and flows.

▶ **Fightmaster Yoga.** The name of this channel may pique your interest. Sorry, it isn't a blend of martial arts and yoga; it's a channel created by yogi Lesley Fightmaster. The videos are aimed at beginner and intermediate levels and include Yoga Fix 90, a ninety-day challenge with a unique practice for each day, in varying styles, with a duration of fifteen to forty minutes per class.

▶ **Gaiam.** The wellness brand, which also has a subscription channel, Gaia.com, offers free YouTube classes like Detox Flow and Restore and Rejuvenate taught by respected instructors such as Rodney Yee and Seane Corn.

▶ **Yoga Journal.** This yoga authority shares yoga pose how-tos, tips on meditation, and sequences geared toward specific interests: climbers, athletes, hip opening, and more.

▶ **The Yogi Matt.** Matt Giordano offers workshops and building-block style sequences to achieve more challenging poses; his handstand strength training video series is key to getting comfortable upside down.

▶ **Yoga with Adriene.** Videos and playlists of varying lengths and styles with specific programs for runners, beginners, travel, weight loss, and more; new videos are posted every Wednesday.

JUST BREATHE

You breathe all day, every day. You don't think about it; you just do it. But do you do it well? There are very few sports in which we are taught how to breathe effectively. And learning to breathe well can be more difficult than it sounds. Yoga is, above all else, breath training. It teaches us to be aware of our breath and to use our breath to overcome difficult or uncomfortable situations.

Throughout class, your teacher may ask, "Are you breathing?" It may sound like a stupid question, but we tend to hold our breath when we're in challenging postures. Yoga trains us to use the breath to find space and calmness in discomfort.

The main breathing technique in yoga is called *ujjayi*, or "breath of victory." You breathe through your nose and fill your lungs completely while slightly contracting your throat. This technique helps calm the mind and relax you while simultaneously warming the body to give you energy. You may hear teachers refer to it as "ocean breathing" because, when done correctly, it should sound like rhythmic ocean waves, rolling in and out. Your breath should be audible to you, but not to the entire room.

My friend Joe likes to joke that a room of new yogis sounds like the entire class is having an orgasm. But if you're grunting, gasping for air, or turning red in the face while doing asanas, it's a sign you need to back off. There's more benefit to sitting back in child's pose and maintaining a steady breath than grunting through another upward dog.

ALTERNATE NOSTRIL BREATHING

If you you're anxious ahead of a race or big meeting, try a few rounds of alternate nostril breathing. The Sanskrit name for this practice, *nadi shodhana*, means "clearing the channels of circulation." When you focus on and deepen your breathing, you'll activate your parasympathetic nervous system, which will calm your mind, slow your heart rate, and reduce your blood pressure. Here's how to practice:

1. Take a comfortable seat and sit tall. Relax your left hand, palm up, in your lap and bring your right hand just in front of your face.

2. Bring the index and middle fingers of your right hand to rest between your eyebrows.

3. Close your eyes and take a deep breath in and out through your nose.

4. Close your right nostril with your right thumb. Inhale through your left nostril slowly and steadily.

5. Close your left nostril with your ring finger so both nostrils are held closed and pause briefly at the top of your inhalation, retaining your breath for a moment.

6. Release your thumb from your right nostril and exhale slowly, then pause briefly at the bottom of your exhalation.

7. Slowly inhale through your right nostril.

8. Close your right nostril with your thumb so both nostrils are held closed and pause briefly.

9. Release your ring finger from your left nostril and exhale slowly through your left nostril, then pause briefly.

10. Repeat for five to ten cycles.

EXPERT ADVICE

(ON THE POWER OF THE BREATH)

I believe the biggest issue for men in yoga today is that they aren't breathing right. Men have to be retrained in how to breathe for yoga. The average American male, especially an athlete or former athlete, has been trained to tighten his abs to attain a six-pack. As a result, men tend to breathe up into their chest but not into their abdomen. Because very few yoga teachers and classes properly emphasize the breath, most men will practice yoga postures in such a way that their breathing gets even more constricted. Couple this with the stress of trying to match the shape of their bodies to the pictures they see in yoga magazines, and it's a recipe for disaster. The problem is that the breath is thrown in and used as a tool to accomplish a pose, instead of the other way around.

—ANDREW TANNER
CHIEF SPOKESPERSON FOR YOGA ALLIANCE AND A BREATH-BASED YOGA INSTRUCTOR

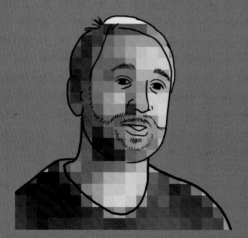

ANDREW TANNER'S KEYS TO MASTERING THE BREATH

Inhalation is for moving up or bending back. Exhalation is for moving down or forward.

Try to keep your breath rate under eight breaths per minute; this will activate the parasympathetic nervous system, bringing a calming quality to your yoga practice.

To breathe, move your transverse abdominals while relaxing your rectus abdominis.

Move slowly, like a sloth, especially during transitions. Slow = strong. Fast = wuss.

Practice slow breath coordinated with seated movements before moving to standing poses.

KAPALABHATI BREATHING

Kapalabhati breathing may feel like blowing snot rockets, but the act of alternating short, explosive exhalations with slightly longer, passive inhalations is actually a deeply detoxifying technique that improves circulation, digestion, and metabolism. Here's how to do it:

1. Take a comfortable seat and sit tall. Relax your left hand, palm up, on your left knee and place your right hand on your stomach so you can feel your abs contract.

2. Take a deep breath and quickly contract the lower belly, pushing a burst of air out of your lungs in a rapid exhalation.

3. Quickly release the contraction and allow your body to inhale automatically and passively.

4. Repeat ten times, focusing on your exhalations.

5. To reset your breathing afterward, breathe deeply for a round or two of the breath.

INVEST IN A GOOD MAT

Clipless bike pedals aren't essential for cycling, but they make it a heck of a lot more efficient. Think of your yoga mat the same way. A mat isn't a must: you can practice on the beach, the carpet, or even a hardwood floor. However, investing in a good mat, just like investing in a pair of clipless bike pedals, enhances performance, especially for beginners. A thin, cheap mat will leave your knees aching in lunges and your back foot sliding in certain poses. You want a mat with some cushion and stickiness.

A lot of mats are made from PVC, which is super harmful for the environment and also reeks of chemicals—not pleasant when your face is squished to the mat during child's pose. Look for mats made from natural rubber, jute, bamboo, organic hemp, or thermoplastic elastomer (TPE). A thicker mat will provide more cushioning but can also weigh up to ten pounds. Yogis on the go may find bulkier mats a pain in the ass to transport from home, to work, to the studio. If you want to use a bulky or heavy mat, ask whether your studio offers mat storage. For a more easily transported option, consider purchasing a travel mat. These are extra thin and light and can be folded (rather than rolled) and stuffed into a bag. In many poses, you can fold a thinner mat if you need more padding. Extra-tall guys don't despair: companies like Manduka make extra-long mats.

If hot yoga is your thing, look for a mat that wicks away moisture, like Gaiam's Studio Select Dry-Grip mat. Another option is to invest in a mat towel, a grippy, highly absorbent towel you can spread over your yoga mat. It will keep your mat dry while also adding traction for sweaty hands and feet. Unlike your yoga mat, you can toss the towel in the wash after each class.

Wiping your mat down after any yoga session is a good, hygienic practice and will also prolong your mat's life. Most studios offer mat cleansing spray, or you can clean it at home with a mixture of equal parts white vinegar and water. As mentioned, germs flourish on yoga mats, especially studio mats. If you're a germaphobe, you'll probably want to purchase yoga mat wipes (yes, that's a thing). Jo-sha's travel-size wipes are made with essential oils and will remove sweat without decreasing the mat's stickiness.

As with any piece of equipment, you have to pay for quality. Expect to spend anywhere from $40 to $150 for a durable mat. The Manduka Pro, considered the Porsche of yoga mats, costs about $130. Anything more expensive, like the $1,000 football-inspired, pebble-grain leather BallerYoga mat, is just indulgent (and ridiculous). Like a baseball glove, a new yoga mat will take a few sessions to break in, and eventually it will wear out. If your mat is starting to crumble, tear, or wear thin, it's time to buy a new one.

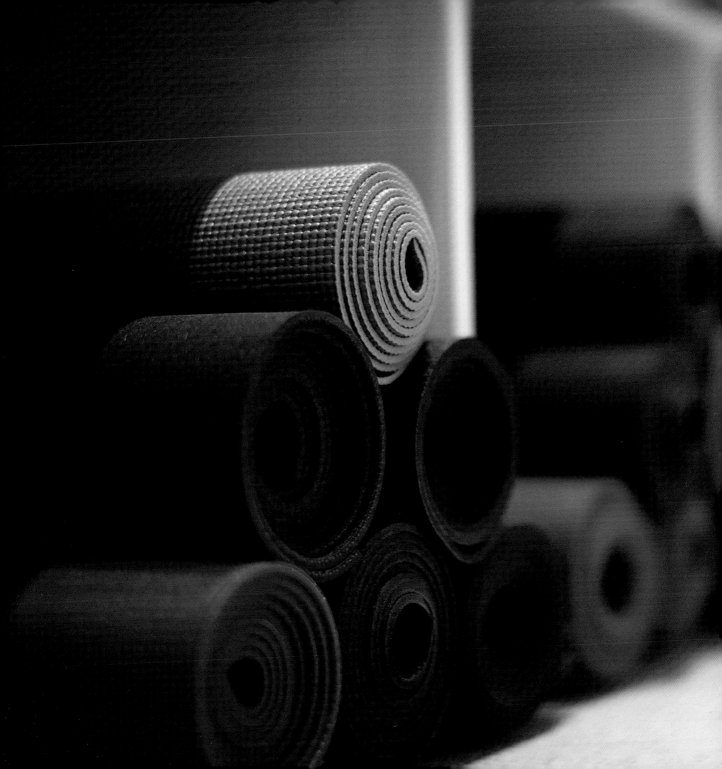

BYO VS STUDIO MATS

Most studios provide complimentary mats or will rent you one for a buck or two. Why, you might wonder, would you bother buying your own and toting it awkwardly from the office to class? For starters, you can never guarantee the cleanliness of a studio mat. It's one thing if your face is smushed into your own sweaty mat, but it's quite another to rest your forehead down where someone else's sweaty feet have been. Studies have shown that yoga mats are perfect incubators for skin infections caused by bacteria, fungi, and viruses. And by investing in your own mat you won't just avoid germs; it can also help you avoid injury if you choose a thickness that's comfortable for your body, especially your wrists and knees. As a final bonus, many studios offer mat storage, so you never need to stress about forgetting your mat at the office or feel self-conscious about lugging it to a post-yoga date.

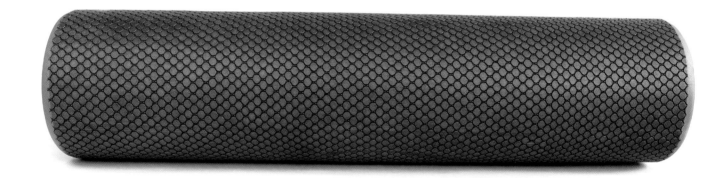

WHAT SHOULD GUYS WEAR TO YOGA?

Despite popular belief (and wildly successful marketing), Lululemon is not yoga's official uniform, and men aren't required to wear a Speedo in Bikram (actually, I beg you, please don't). Yoga is about comfort. If you feel ridiculous in spandex, there's no need to go there. If you feel self-conscious with your shirt off, keep it on—even if it is drenched in sweat. You don't have to spend a lot of money on fancy clothing made from organic, sustainable, fair-trade cotton sourced from Kyrgyzstan and blessed by a monk. That old T-shirt that you wear to the gym will do just fine.

What matters most when it comes to clothing isn't the brand or the colors but the fit. You want clothing that makes it easy for teachers to see how your body is aligned, from feet to shoulder blades, so they can adjust your pose, so avoid baggy basketball shorts. Also avoid extra-short shorts that will give the room a free peep show when you do a forward fold. (A friend of mine made the mistake of wearing short running shorts to Bikram and ended up lying in *savasana* for half the class because his balls kept falling out when he bent over in downward dog.) Board shorts are actually ideal yoga wear for guys—manly, yet functional.

EXPERT ADVICE

(ON INVERSIONS)

Inversions improve proprioception, or awareness of your body in space. When you become aware of your body in space and then flip upside down, your relationship to gravity changes and your ability to sense where your body is in space becomes much greater. The steps to handstand (page 148) are actually pretty simple. It's like anything else: You have to break something big down into small steps that are easy and accessible. Once you understand and master the small steps, that big thing will become approachable. Here are the small steps involved in handstand.

—MATT GIORDANO
YOGA INSTRUCTOR

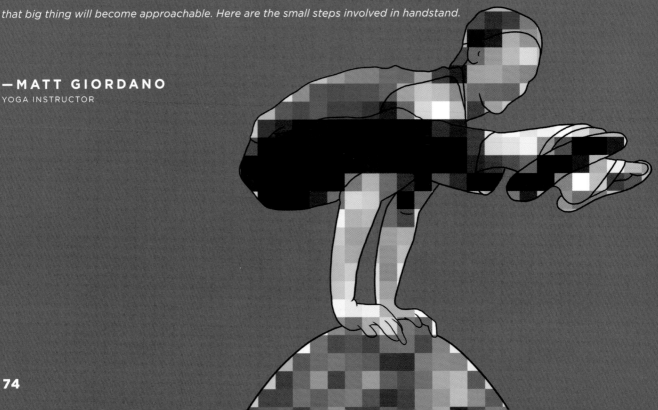

MATT GIORDANO'S KEYS TO MASTERING HANDSTAND

Develop finger, wrist, and hand strength. Balancing in handstand is nothing more than leaning your body weight into your fingers and your fingers resisting that body weight. Work on that feeling of resistance first on your hands and knees, then in plank pose (page 156), then in downward dog (page 138), and eventually in arm balances like crow (right, page 136).

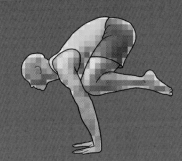

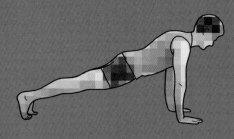

Develop push strength. Push strength comes from elevating your scapula, or honing your military press muscles. When you raise a barbell overhead, you push it up and extend until your elbows are straight. If you're working your full range of motion, your trapezius muscles should fire as your shoulders go up toward your ears. That's the reach and push you'll feel in handstand. Practice honing push strength in plank pose (left, page 156).

Be willing to use the wall. Using the wall won't help you structurally, but it will help you get over any mental fear of being upside down or falling. Hold the pose against the wall to get used to what it feels like to have your body inverted. For more advanced practice, face your belly to the wall and use the wall to help with alignment rather than balance. Have a teacher show you how to safely cartwheel out of the pose before you start trying handstand in the middle of the room.

MAD PROPS

Asking for help or requesting assistance, whether at work or in sports, is often viewed as a sign of weakness or lack of athleticism. Not so in yoga. B. K. S. Iyengar introduced the use of props in yoga so that everyone—no matter their age, flexibility, height, weight, or fitness level—could safely access the benefits of postures. Props allow anyone, even people working with an injury, to find correct alignment, stretch more deeply, and relax into a pose. If you've ever found yourself straining and grunting as you attempted to clasp your hands behind your back in cow face, even as your teacher said, "Relax and breathe deeply into the pose," next time try grabbing a strap in either hand. You'll realize your teacher isn't a sadist.

For many beginners, yoga is about the end point: the finish line is touching their toes or clasping their hands behind their back. You won't make any gains with this attitude. If you think a successful revolved triangle pose means placing your hand on the floor, you're missing the point. The point of revolved triangle isn't to touch your hand to the floor; it's to stretch your IT band and the muscles on the side of your hip. If you compromise the pose by reaching for the floor, you take the stretch off of these places. And if you don't have the range of motion needed to touch the floor, you'll end up jutting your hip out to the side, compressing your lower back, and crunching your sacroiliac (SI) joint. But hey, your hand reached the ground, right?

Some people may try to tell you that using props is cheating, but not using props is cheating yourself out of the real benefits of yoga. Even the most experienced practitioners gain benefits from using a little extra support.

Also, be aware that male and female bodies are anatomically different—and not just in the obvious ways. Don't get discouraged if every girl in the room is seated cross-legged in easy pose with her knees resting on the ground while your knees are up in your armpits. For this pose, most men need to sit on a block or a folded blanket in order to find a comfortable pelvic tilt. Similarly, sitting with your hips raised will make any seated forward fold more comfortable. Or if you find yourself struggling to step your leg through from downward dog to warrior 1, try placing your hands on blocks. The extra height will make it easier until you've developed the range of motion necessary to do the move unassisted.

As with yoga apparel, you'll find that you can purchase a wide array of props—blocks, bolsters, straps, and so on—color coordinated if you're into that. But there are many DIY options as well. You could use a phone book in place of a block to sit on, or a twisted T-shirt to wrap around the soles of your feet, instead of a strap, to tug on and help you bend into forward fold.

Blocks. Most yoga studios offer a variety of blocks made from either foam, cork, or wood. Many people choose their blocks based on aesthetics, but the various materials actually offer different benefits. Foam blocks provide more cushioning. They aren't as stable, but they contour to the shape of our bones. For example, if you're doing a more restorative practice, you may want a softer block to place under your sacrum. Or if you're working toward half front splits, you might feel like your groin is going to tear. Placing a soft block (or two) under your pelvis will allow you to slowly and hopefully painlessly sink into your most comfortable version of the pose. A harder block, made from cork or wood, is a great tool for stability or extra lift in balancing poses or backbends. Beginners may find that placing sturdier blocks beneath their hands will give them more space to step through to crescent lunge, for examples, or give them more height to get into crow pose.

Blocks don't just assist in bridging the gap between you and the floor; they can also help you keep your muscles engaged. You may find it helpful to squeeze a foam block between your thighs in bridge to keep your knees in line with the hips and ensure that your adductors are firing. Blocks can also be used as spacers to set up the proper foundation of a pose. If you can't picture what your teacher means when he or she says "keep your elbows under your shoulders" in dolphin pose, place a block between them as a reminder. Most blocks are 4 by 6 by 9 inches, so they can be placed at three different heights (flat, on edge, or on end), allowing you to use the different levels to slowly work your way into a pose until you no longer need the assistance of props.

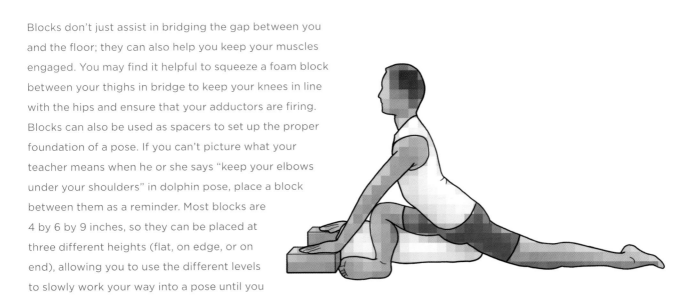

Blanket. How the traditional woven Mexican blanket became the go-to blanket for yogis is a mystery, but you'll find stacks of them at your studio. If you're practicing at home and don't have one, you can use any thick blanket or even bath towels. A blanket is useful for bringing the floor closer or for cushioning.

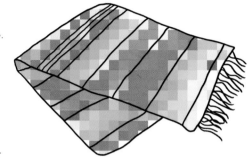

Learning to properly roll or fold a yoga blanket may initially seem like mastering origami, but it's important to get it right. You want the rolled or folded blanket to have clean edges and be free of creases and lumps so it provides smooth, stable, comfortable support for your body. Start by mastering the foundation. Open the blanket and smooth out the creases. Fold the blanket in half lengthwise, to form a narrower rectangle. Then fold it in half in the other direction, bringing the two fringed ends together. Fold once more in the same way.

Rolled or folded, a blanket can provide extra support during forward folds, twists, and chest openers. If you have sensitive knees, try placing a blanket beneath your knees in kneeling poses like table, cat and cow, or camel. In seated postures, a folded blanket can help raise your hips and tilt your pelvis forward. Or if your hips are tight, you can place a blanket under your glutes to help open your hips in poses like pigeon. Some teachers will ask if you want to be covered with a blanket as you settle into *savasana*, to keep your body warm so you can relax. If the thought of draping a communal blanket across your body grosses you out, bring an extra layer, like a sweatshirt or long-sleeved shirt, to put on during *savasana*.

Bolster. Think of a bolster as a body pillow. The long, rectangular cushion is meant to support part of your body so you can simultaneously relax and open more deeply into a pose. Bolsters are key props in restorative and Iyengar classes. Simply lying with a bolster aligned under your head, shoulders, and spine will open up your chest while also stretching the diaphragm and abdominals and improving digestion. Lying with a bolster lengthwise beneath your back during *savasana* or beneath your lower back in legs up the wall pose (right) will help you release more deeply into relaxation, or placing a bolster under your knees in *savasana* will create more space in your lower back and relieve any lower back tension.

Placing a bolster directly in front of you in wide-angle seated forward fold or even seated forward fold allows you to rest in the pose if your chest and stomach can't reach your legs or the ground. If you're practicing at home, you can improvise with a long, firm cushion, like a couch cushion.

Strap or belt. Belts help stabilize the joints and create traction and space in compressed, inflexible parts of the body. You might think of a strap as giving you Go-Go Gadget arms, as it puts your toes within reach. So if your feet seem miles away in seated forward fold, loop a strap around the soles of your feet and activate your legs as you gently tug the straps to hinge forward. If you have tight shoulders, as many guys do, you probably won't be able to clasp your hands behind your back in poses like cow face, at least not initially. In that case, a strap will be your best friend, allowing you to open up into poses while keeping your spine long and chest lifted. Using a strap as you start to work on bound poses, like bound extended side angle, allows the chest to open without sacrificing the integrity of the pose.

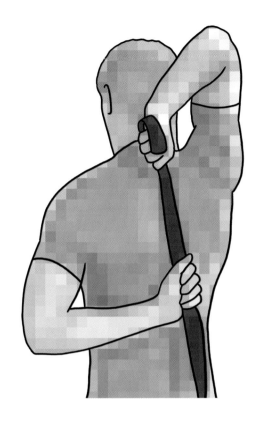

If you're a beginner, you'll find that a strap provides great guidance for staying in proper alignment and also serves as a helpful reminder to keep your muscles engaged. For example, looping a strap around your thighs, just above your knees, in mountain pose, chair pose, or plank pose will help you activate your thigh muscles and quads, which will prevent your knees from rolling inward. Or you can place a looped strap around your arms, just above your elbows, to keep your elbows from splaying outward and to keep your arms engaged as you work on poses like forearm plank or dolphin. When using the strap in these ways, you want the loop to be bracing, so you feel tension when you push out against it, but not so tight that it cuts off circulation.

A strap also helps in balancing poses, like extended hand to big toe pose. Most people fall out of alignment, jutting their hip out and letting their chest sink as they reach for the toe. Looping a strap around the foot provides traction that aids in balance and also allows you to maintain a straight spine and level hips.

Wedge: Because men tend to be tighter in the hips, you may need to use a prop to ensure good body mechanics in seated forward folds. Sitting on a block or bolster can help by lifting you up, but sitting on a downward slope will allow for an anterior pelvic title so you can more easily hinge forward. Although you can fold a blanket into a sloped shape, it's generally more effective to use a wedge, which is a long, doorstop-shaped foam prop that can be placed under the sitting bones to help initiate a more comfortable forward fold. Wedges are also great for people who suffer from carpal tunnel syndrome or weak wrists, who might experience pain during weight-bearing exercises that require flat palms. To take pressure off of the wrists, orient the wedge sloping down toward the front of the mat and place the knuckles of the hands on the mat and the heel of the hand on downward slope of the wedge.

EXPERT ADVICE

(ON INJURY PREVENTION)

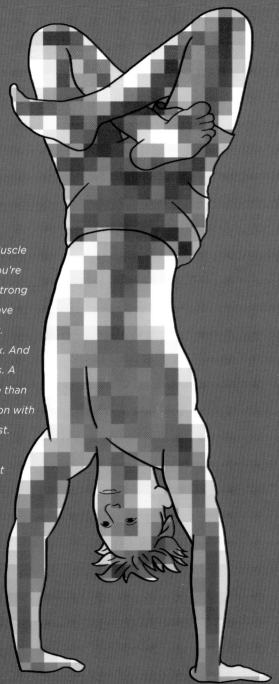

Everyone talks about how good yoga is for you, but it can also hurt you. Muscle limits your range of motion, so if you try to muscle your way into poses, you're likely to get injured. Most men are strong in the upper body. They have a strong chest, arms, and shoulders, so arm balances are easy. But because they have limited mobility in their chest and shoulders, backbends are really difficult. When men try to do backbends, the load often ends up in their lower back. And when the hips are tight—and most men's are—the load goes into the knees. A yoga pose in which the load isn't distributed properly in the joints is worse than a jujitsu submission hold. Yoga requires you to have a two-way conversation with your nervous system. You need to listen to your bodily feedback and adjust.

Don't get dejected if you can't do a pose without the assistance or support of props. I remember my teacher in Hawaii looking at me trying to do a split and saying, "If you practice that every day, you'll get it in twenty years." I was like, "That long to get my crotch on the floor?!" That moment created a big shift in my perspective. The goal isn't to get your crotch on the floor; it's to leave the practice feeling better than when you walked in, not injured because of your ego.

—EOIN FINN
FOUNDER OF BLISSOLOGY YOGA

MUSIC VS NO MUSIC

Purists argue that yoga is a moving meditation, not a dance. Music, especially music with lyrics, can disrupt focus and concentration, two of yoga's main principles. But yoga doesn't have to be super serious—it can and should be fun. Music motivates us, enhances mood, and can help us find our flow. Just as you might gravitate to a spinning instructor with a great playlist, you could find yourself gravitating to a yoga instructor based on what's on his or her iPod. In addition to the common new-age soundtracks, there are teachers who play '80s classics, techno beats, and even heavy metal during class. Some teachers choreograph entire classes to a single artist, like the Grateful Dead, or instruct classes to the beat of a live DJ. A few may even play a guitar or an Indian harmonium at the start and end of class. Just one caveat: If you're a beginner, be aware that music can make it challenging to hear the instructor and to tune in to your breath. If you practice to music at home, remember that yoga isn't a dance. You want to follow the rhythm of your breath, not a beat.

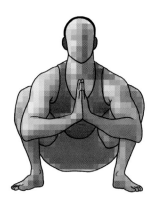

EXPERT ADVICE

(ON THE POWER OF MUSIC)

Throughout my life I've developed a love and compassion for creative music solely based on my emotional response. The beats moved me. The melodies grooved me. The lyrics soothed me. I wanted to share these feelings with the world. My ambition in creating vinyasa flow music mix projects is to use the journey of music to tap into people's collective memory so they can grow into their greatest potential by overcoming fears and moving beyond their past. Music has the power to take us places. It evokes so much emotion; it is the path to the heart no matter who you are.

—TYLER LAMBUTH, AKA DJ BHAKTI STYLER
YOGA INSTRUCTOR AND DJ AT ASPEN SHAKTI SHALA

CHAPTER 5

WHEN YOGA?

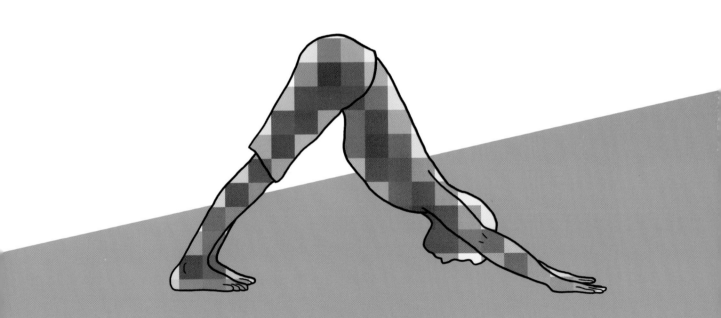

DOES TIME OF DAY MATTER?

If we were all virtuous yogis, we would match our mealtimes, bedtime, and yoga practice to the ayurvedic clock. This age-old timepiece breaks the day into six, four-hour chunks, with one daytime chunk and one nighttime chunk being assigned to each of the three *doshas*, or mind-body types. The earthy, grounding *kapha dosha* reigns from 6 a.m. to 10 a.m.; the hot, fiery *pitta dosha* from 10 a.m. to 2 p.m.; and the light, airy *vata dosha* from 2 p.m. until 6 p.m. And then the cycle begins again. In a perfect ayurvedic world, we'd start our yoga practice at sunrise, a peaceful time of day when our circadian rhythm starts awakening the body. We'd eat our biggest meal of the day in the afternoon, when our fiery *pitta dosha* is fueling our metabolism. And by 6 p.m., we'd be winding down from our day, quieting the mind and body in preparation for rest.

I know very few people, other than monks or swamis, who can keep such a schedule in modern society. The reality is that, for most of us, our clock revolves around work and family. And then there are personal inclinations: some of us are morning people and others are night owls. Yoga, like any other physical practice, is personal, and the best way to find out what time of day is ideal for your body, mind, and schedule is to experiment.

All of that said, you may find it helpful to know that some styles of yoga (vinyasa) and certain postures (backbends) are more invigorating, while other styles (yin) and postures (forward folds) are calming. Consider what you want to get from the practice and incorporate that into your decision about when to practice, keeping your own needs in mind. You may find that an energizing 6 a.m. vinyasa flow class pumps you up to start your day, or your body might be too stiff to bend into standing forward fold or hinge into extended triangle first thing in the morning. At lunchtime, a hatha yoga class might reset your mind for the rest of the day, whereas a restorative yin class might put you in nap mode. And a 7 p.m. power yoga class may be a perfect fit for you, or it might prevent you from falling asleep at night. In short, the perfect time for yoga is the time that works best for you.

HOW LONG AND HOW OFTEN TO PRACTICE?

Most studios offer classes that range from sixty to ninety minutes. Not all of us have that much time every day, but that doesn't mean we can't benefit from yoga. It's more valuable to practice for fifteen minutes and be fully present than to practice for sixty minutes while glancing at your smartphone. It's just like any other workout: you can slog away on the elliptical machine for an hour while answering emails and watching ESPN, or you can crank out twenty minutes of intervals. When it comes to exercise, something is always better than nothing, and you'll always get a bigger return for your efforts when you give 100 percent.

In yoga, much like running, you build up mental and physical endurance over time. Jumping right into a ninety-minute Bikram class can feel like attempting a marathon with zero training. Ease into the practice by setting attainable goals. For example, devote ten minutes to yoga three days a week for a month. Then, the next month, bump it to twenty minutes. Or rather than committing to taking one class per week, choose one pose to incorporate into your day-to-day routine, like legs up the wall after a long run, or seated cat and cow at your desk. Yoga doesn't have to be a marriage; you can gain huge benefits from the occasional fling.

START YOUR DAY BY SALUTING THE SUN

Sun salutation A (*surya namaskar* A) is a simple series often used to warm up the body in studio classes. It's also easy to practice at home. The sequence of eight postures is often performed in sets of five, but if you're new to the practice, start with two or three and gradually work your way up to more repetitions. Remember to let the breath lead the movement. Each inhalation and each exhalation should draw you into and through the next pose.

1. Begin by standing in mountain pose (page 154) with your feet hip-width apart and your weight distributed evenly over both feet. Press your palms in prayer position at your heart and establish your *ujjayi* breath (page 66).

2. As you inhale, stretch your arms to the sides and overhead into upward salute (page 175). Gently arch your back as you reach your heart and arms to the ceiling.

3. As you exhale, fold from the hips into standing forward fold (page 168), keeping your legs engaged. Bend your knees if necessary and rest your hands beside your feet.

4. As you inhale, lengthen your spine forward into standing half forward fold (page 169). The spine is extended and the gaze lifted. Your fingertips can be on the floor or rise to your shins.

5. As you exhale, step or lightly hop your feet back into plank pose (page 156). Take a full breath in to lengthen your body out through your heels.

6. Exhaling, lower slowly into *chaturanga* (page 145).

7. Inhaling, slide your chest forward and straighten your arms into upward dog (page 174), with the tops of your feet pressing against the floor. Draw your shoulders back and open your chest.

8. Exhaling, roll over your feet, tuck your toes under and press back into downward dog (page 138). Hold this position for five breaths.

9. On your fifth exhalation, bend your knees and look between your hands. Then, as you inhale, step or lightly hop your feet between your hands, returning to standing half forward fold.

10. Exhaling, release into standing forward fold.

11. Inhaling, reach your arms out to your sides and, with a back flat, come to an upright standing position, extending your arms overhead in upward salute.

12. Exhaling, return to mountain and bring your hands to prayer position at your heart.

13. Repeat.

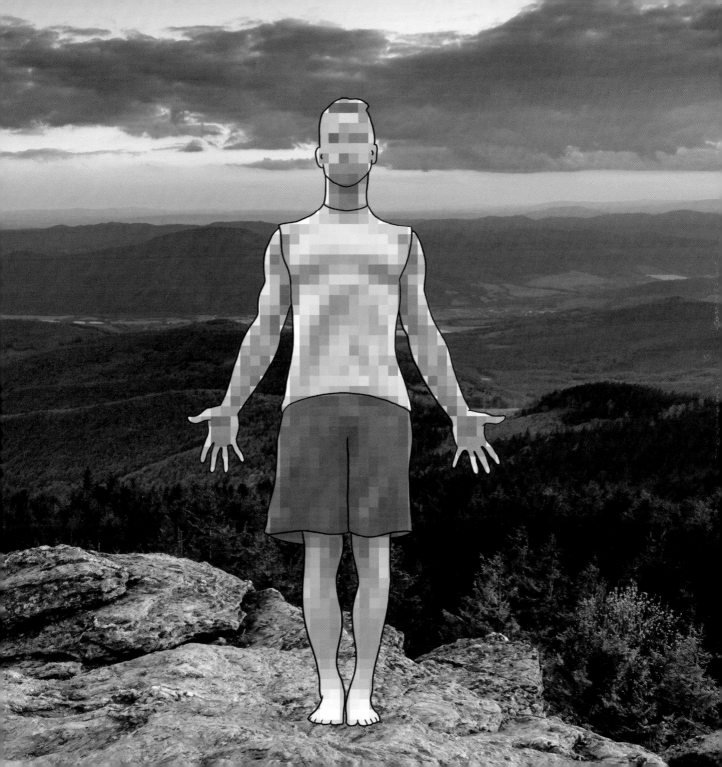

JEFF KRASNO & SEAN HOESS

COFOUNDERS OF WANDERLUST

I was exposed to yoga through my wife (and now business partner), Schuyler Grant. Her yoga studio was literally above my office in Tribeca. Even though yoga has been around me for more than twenty years, it wasn't until recently, when my body started breaking down, that I integrated it into my life. I'd always been an athlete, and suddenly my body couldn't do what it used to be able to do. I rarely go to a studio and take a ninety-minute class, but I do weave yoga into my workouts and my workday. I might do a couple of sun salutations at the gym or after a run. I have low back pain, so I try to do lower back strengthening poses, like hero pose (virasana). Sometimes I sit on a block in hero pose, prop up my computer in front of me, and work like that for forty-five minutes. I also incorporate poses into my sports. Chair pose has become my return serve stance in tennis. I also do this silly thing called joga, which is a mix of running and yoga. I keep my torso and back very upright and go through warrior one and warrior two poses while jogging. I'm sure I look ridiculous, but it lets me get in some chest and shoulder opening while working on cardio on the trails. I also have a routine I do in the sauna.

I am an occasional yogi surrounded by hard-core yogis, mostly women. Jeff and I used to be in the music business, and Jeff's wife, Schuyler, was running yoga trips to Costa Rica. I thought, "Yoga be damned, I'll go for the jungle, ocean, and surf." I actually enjoyed the yoga piece but never became a regular. Yoga is the hardest physical thing I have ever done in my life. I'm used to playing sports, and if you think about it, in almost every single sport a man can have some strength or power advantage over a woman. We can usually throw harder, kick farther, run faster. Not so in yoga. The average woman is better at yoga than the average man, and it's intimidating going into this world where you're in the minority and everyone around you is doing better than you. No man wants to be in a room full of hot women and be seen grunting and sweating and struggling. This is the rare occasion where a man's strength works against him. Your muscles are so tight they oppose every single thing the teacher instructs you to do. It's incredibly humbling.

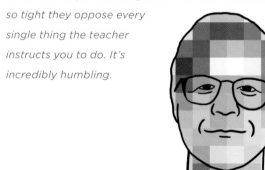

CAN YOU PRACTICE ON A FULL STOMACH?

Drinking beer and napping are about the only two things that should be practiced on a full stomach. As with running, swimming, or any other form of physical exercise, it's best to avoid doing yoga immediately after a meal. One of the reasons yoga devotees tout an early morning practice is because the stomach is at its emptiest when we wake. In yoga, we twist side to side, bend forward and backward, and turn upside down. If you just ate a cheeseburger, balancing on your belly in locust pose is going to cause serious discomfort. A good rule of thumb is to eat at least two to three hours before class. If you're starving, opt for something light, like nuts, fruit, or juice, at least thirty minutes before class.

CAN YOU DRINK BEER AFTER YOGA?

The detox-retox concept has become incredibly popular, adding a social, boozy element to activities like cycling, running, and, yes, even yoga. Beer before or during yoga is definitely a bad idea. But a cold beer after yoga is a nice reward. Some yoga groups, like Hoppy Yoga in San Diego, host classes at breweries, followed by a beer social. Yoga retreats, like those put on by Surf Yoga Beer in Costa Rica, Nicaragua, and other exotic locations, promote balancing a healthy lifestyle with a bit of indulgence. That said, after any class it's best to drink at least six ounces of water before sipping a brew. If you've just finished a hot yoga class, reach for electrolyte-enhanced water or coconut water so you can rehydrate before slamming a beer. And it's probably best to order a low-alcohol session beer, like a kölsch, rather than a high-octane double IPA.

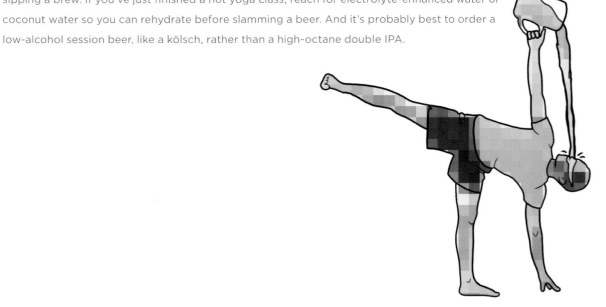

WHAT'S THE DEAL WITH SAVASANA?

Savasana, aka corpse pose (page 132), is the final posture done at the end of class to seal your practice. Unlike balancing on one leg in tree pose or backbending in locust, *savasana* requires you to do nothing more than lie down, close your eyes, and relax. Yet it's often called the hardest pose in yoga. If you've ever practiced yoga in a studio, you've probably experienced the end of class exodus prior to *savasana*—or maybe you've been part of it. You've just opened your hamstrings and back and broke a sweat doing a seemingly never-ending series of sun salutations (page 88) and then the teacher asks you to lie down and do nothing for a few minutes. This seems like the perfect opportunity for time-crunched yogis to sneak out of class early and beat the locker room rush. But if you do that, you'll miss the best part of the practice. An instructor once told me that yoga without *savasana* is like sex without an orgasm. (That might be an extreme comparison, but you get the point).

Savasana is the culmination of the practice, a time when all of the benefits of yoga settle in. When we lie in *savasana*, any mental or physical stress we were holding on to gets released. Heart rate slows, blood pressure drops, and tension melts away. And as relaxing as that sounds, stopping the mind from racing is difficult and makes this pose incredibly hard to master. Quieting the mind and body are things we rarely do in our day-to-day lives (except when we sleep).

Finally, don't be afraid of nodding off—or snoring! The intention of *savasana* is to relax with attention. But if you do fall asleep, it just means that your body and mind have reached a state of complete relaxation. Someone will eventually wake you up.

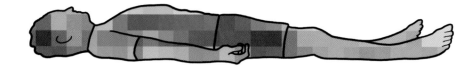

BEDTIME YOGA

If your mind is racing as you head to bed, try integrating a few yoga poses into your evening routine; the combination of breath and movement will help quiet the mind. Restorative postures can be particularly helpful for combating stress and insomnia. Use as many props as possible for more support and deeper relaxation.

1. Begin in child's pose (page 130).

2. Rise to hands and knees and flow through a few sequences of cat and cow (page 128).

3. Press back to downward dog (page 138).

4. Step your right leg through to lizard pose (page 152) and hold for a few rounds of breath. Step your right leg back to plank pose, flow through *chaturanga* (page 145) to upward dog (page 174) then exhale and press back into downward dog. Hold for one round of breath. Then step your left leg through to lizard pose and repeat the sequence.

5. Lie down onto your back for reclining butterfly (page 158).

6. From reclining butterfly, bring your knees back up, stretch your legs forward, and then move into plow pose (page 157).

7. End in a sleepy *savasana* (page 132).

CHAPTER 6

WHERE YOGA?

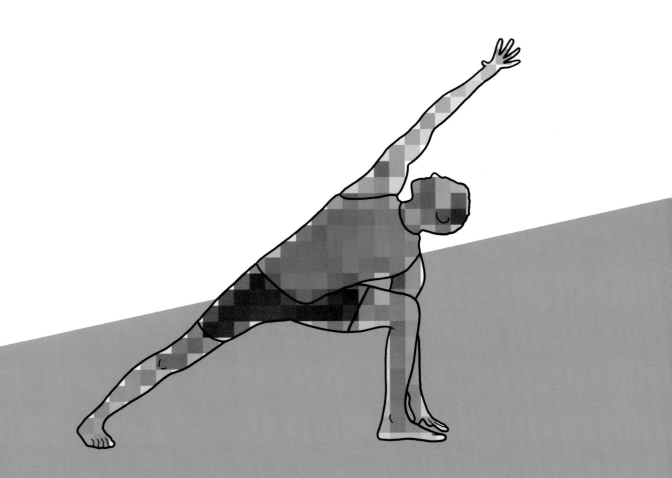

HOW TO CHOOSE A STUDIO

Choosing a yoga studio is kind of like choosing a gym. Cost and convenience are two major considerations. You can spend hundreds of dollars to belong to a shiny modern studio with a locker room and juice bar, or you can find a donation-based studio, like Yoga to the People. As you explore your options, don't feel pressured into committing to a membership. Most studios have the option to pay a drop-in fee, and many offer discounts or deals for new students.

What truly matters is finding a studio where you connect with a teacher (see page 64) and where the class schedule fits with your own. Also, if you have a preferred style of yoga (see page 54), look for a studio that offers that type of class. For example, if you know that you're a power yogi, you may want to join a power yoga–specific studio, like CorePower. If, on the other hand, you're still figuring out your style, look for studios that offer a variety of classes at a variety of levels. Also consider your personality. If you like the social aspect of the gym, you might want a yoga studio that offers a similar sense of community. Of course, if you already have a gym membership, ask whether they offer yoga, then see if any of the classes and instructors click with you.

You might also consider logistics. For example, if you travel for work, you might want to look into a studio chain, such as YogaWorks or Jivamukti Yoga, with memberships that offer access to a country-wide, and sometimes international, network of studios.

CLASS LEVEL MATTERS

Most studios have classes labeled "beginner's" or "level 1" that focus on mastering foundational poses. Classes labeled "level 2," "level 3," or "advanced" are geared toward experienced yogis who already understand the basic terminology and fundamental postures. Many studios offer "open level" or "all level" classes, where the experience of students can vary widely. In these mixed-level classes, the teacher is there to guide the practice with students adjusting to their own comfort level.

If you've ever accidentally ended up in the six-minute-mile corral instead of the eleven-minute-mile corral at a 5K race, that's kind of how you'll feel if you're a beginner in a level 2 to 3 vinyasa class. Yoga classes have designated levels for a reason. A roomful of yogis dropping into *chaturanga* from handstand can be intimidating if you're not even sure how to do child's pose. If you're a beginner, you'll definitely want to start out in beginner-level or slow flow classes so you can master the basic postures in proper alignment, learn to breathe correctly, and get a handle on yoga terminology.

If you accidentally (or overambitiously) find yourself in an advanced class, check your ego at the door, keep your focus on yourself rather than the pretzel-twisted yogi next to you, and let your breath dictate how far to push yourself.

WHAT LEVEL ARE YOU?

Level 1	Level 2	Level 3
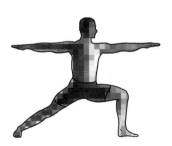	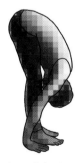	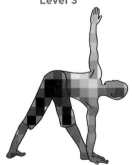
You can't remember the difference between warrior 2 and warrior 3 and stop breathing in extended triangle.	You feel confident moving through sun salutation A on your own but still haven't mastered arm balances like crow and inversions like headstand.	You've mastered the foundational poses and can breathe deeply and evenly in challenging poses like revolved triangle.

STUDIO ETIQUETTE

It's normal to feel a bit clueless when walking into your first yoga class. These tips will help you avoid a major studio faux pas. And if you still feel self-conscious after reading them, remember: there's no judgment in yoga.

Turn off your phone. Yoga is about minimizing distractions. You may initially experience separation anxiety, but after a few classes you'll start looking forward to disconnecting for an hour.

If you arrive a few minutes late and the entire class is already seated and chanting "om," wait until opening meditation has finished, then quietly tiptoe into class, spread out your mat, and start following along. If you need to warm up, spend a few minutes pedaling your feet in downward dog before joining the flow.

If you have to leave early, tell your teacher before class begins and take a seat close to the exit. Be as stealthy as possible when leaving the room so as not to disrupt other students. And don't jump up and run out the door when the teacher says its time for *savasana*—that's just rude.

Clean up after yourself. If you've borrowed props, return them in a respectable manner; for example, fold your blanket neatly rather than stuffing it onto the shelf. If you're using a studio mat and there's a sheen of sweat on it, wipe it off, then spray it with disinfectant. There are few things worse than unrolling a damp, stinky mat.

Farts happen, especially when we twist our bodies into detoxifying poses. My brother used to say that it's funnier when girls fart. Try not to giggle. You'll know you've achieved a Zen-like state when you can maintain tree pose, unwavering, when the girl next to you lets one rip.

It's okay to take time out, and even encouraged. There's no shame in doing cobra instead of upward dog if your lower back is aching and your wrists are throbbing. If you're having an off day or just feel tired after a challenging pose, sit back in child's pose. You're not admitting defeat; you're accepting your body's limitations on that particular day.

If you're uncomfortable with the chanting, even if it's a simple opening "om," no one will judge you—or probably even notice—if you sit in silence. Lip-syncing is the next step, and eventually you may find yourself quietly humming along.

Questions are encouraged, but ask them before or after class. Of course, teachers aren't mind readers, so if you have an injury or other limitation, let the teacher know before class. And if a pose felt uncomfortable or a cue was confusing, pull your teacher aside after class to discuss it.

Yoga is not a competition. Avoid comparing your pose to that of the person next to you—or worse, judging the person next to you. I once had a friend loudly point out, "That buff dude is doing *chaturanga* on his knees. What a pussy!" You may think it, but you don't have to voice it.

Avoid making observations about your own practice. In one class, the guy next to me shouted out, "I just nailed tree pose. Booyah!" If you have a breakthrough, cheer yourself internally. If you want to boast, you can do that after class.

Be mindful of personal space. Class may get crowded, but no one wants a sweaty ass in his or her face. And if the studio is packed, that probably isn't the time to attempt your first headstand.

Don't check yourself out in the mirror. The mirror is there for you to check your alignment, not your hair.

Breathe deeply but quietly. Your breathing shouldn't make you sound like a porn star.

Don't stink. Avoid loading up on cologne before class and try to use a deodorant that actually works.

YOGA WORKSHOPS:
NOT JUST FOR ADVANCED YOGIS

You may see flyers in your studio promoting weekend, weeklong, or even multiweek workshops. These programs can be a great way to fine-tune aspects of your practice in a more intensive setting. For beginners, the common refrain in regular classes is not to push too far or to back off if a pose feels too intense. But in order to advance, you need to push yourself—safely—toward the next level of a pose. Some workshops focus on specific aspects of the physical form, like inversions or arm balances, while others focus on the breath or more spiritual aspects. Those with a physical focus often break down elements of poses and help participants build strength and develop technique to promote proper alignment in more challenging postures.

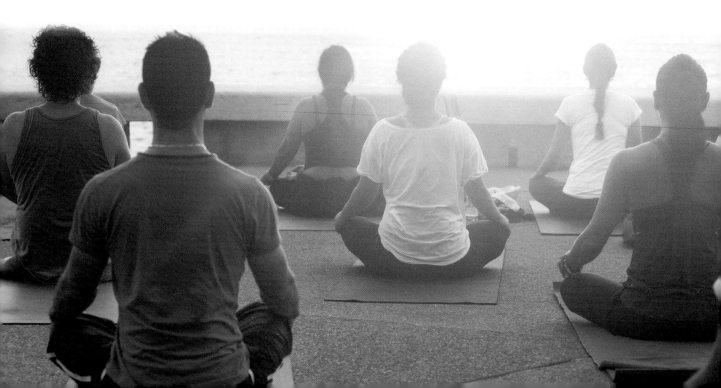

EXPERT ADVICE

(ON DEVELOPING A HOME PRACTICE)

When practicing at home, remember to do things to mobilize all ranges of the spine and the major range of motion in the hips. Technically, there are six ranges of motion for the spinal column, but they can really be boiled down to four: side bending, back bending, forward bending, and twisting. During home practice, be sure to choose a posture out of each of these four categories to ensure your spine has full mobility. There are hundreds of variations to choose from in order to work the full range of motion. For example, you could string together a reverse warrior (page 160) for a side bend, upward dog (page 174) for a backbend, standing forward fold (page 168) for a forward bend, and revolved chair (page 161) for a twist. For the hips, you want to address the outer hips and inner thighs. A classic outer hip stretch is pigeon (page 155). Anything that stretches the groin will work the inner hips, like butterfly (page 125).

—DAVID MAGONE
FOUNDER OF PRANAVAYU YOGA

YOGA IN THE BEDROOM

The best sex I've ever had has been with men who do yoga. I'm not talking guys who perform Cirque du Soleil–style bedroom theatrics, just men who are more focused, attentive, and in tune with their body and breath. Research suggests that *pranayama*, the breathing techniques used in yoga, release the same chemicals in the brain as sex does, so more time on the mat may make for better sex.

Postures like chair (page 129), wide-angle seated forward fold (page 179), and bridge (page 124) increase blood flow to the pelvic region, which can stimulate a sexual response. Yoga also allows us to become more comfortable with vulnerability—both on the mat and between the sheets. Of course, added flexibility won't hurt your bedroom antics either.

Think of yoga as the ultimate foreplay. There are plenty of sensually oriented books and DVDs on tantric yoga that will wow you with new positions to try with your lover. Or you can try something as simple as the following three poses.

Hand to heart pose. Lie together with your partner, one of you on your back and the other lying alongside, propped on one arm. Look into each other's eyes, and each place the palm of one hand over the other's heart. Feel each other's heartbeat, then focus on breathing slowly and in unison. The pose may sound cheesy, but it's intensely intimate and will deepen the connection you have with each other.

Seated spinal twist. Sit cross-legged with your partner, back-to-back. As each of you turns your head and torso to the right, reach for the other's left thigh with your right hand, and your own right thigh with your left hand. You can deepen the twist by pulling on each other's thigh. Try to slow and synchronize your breathing.

Seated forward fold with backbend. This chest, back, and hamstring opener requires trust and some balance to do as a pair. Sit back-to-back, with your legs straight out in front of you and your partner's knees bent and feet flat on the floor. As you fold forward, your partner leans back against you. Once you're stable, your partner extends the arms overhead as you reach for your toes. To go deeper into the pose, reach for your partner's wrists and pull your partner more deeply into the stretch.

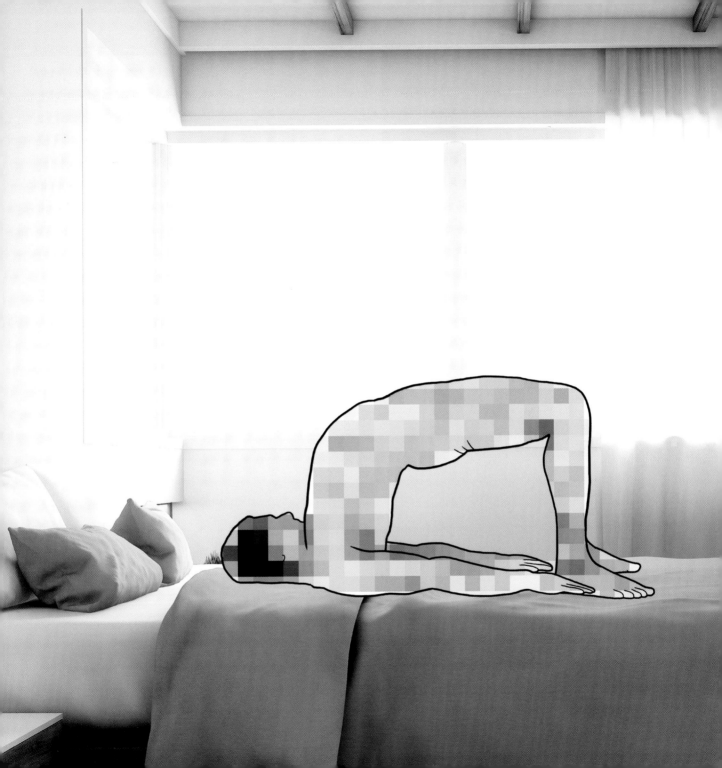

YOGA AT WORK

For too many of us, our aches and pains aren't from the basketball court or the soccer field; they're from long hours logged at the office. The majority of us spend our days sitting hunched over a computer. As a result, we suffer low back pain, tight hips, stiff wrists and neck, and tense shoulders. You can undo the damage of a desk job by integrating yoga into your workday. This doesn't mean you have to unfurl a mat in your cubicle. Simply doing few simple stretches at your desk can help open up your body; it can also calm your mind before a meeting or presentation.

FIVE DESK POSES

1. The arm position of eagle (page 139) can counterbalance shoulder and neck strain from sitting in front of a computer.

2. You can do seated twist (page 165) while sitting in your office chair to release muscles in your back that stiffen after you've been stuck in a seated position for hours.

3. You can open up your spine with a gentle seated backbend. On an inhalation, reach your arms up to the ceiling and open them wide. As you exhale, extend your back and upper chest up and over the back of your chair.

4. Use your desk to help open up tight shoulders. Stand a few feet from your desk, then hinge at your hips, touching your hands to the edge of your desk until you form a 90-degree angle. Drop your head and chest between your arms to stretch the shoulders.

5. Open up tight hip flexors with seated pigeon pose (page 155). While seated in your chair with both feet flat on the floor, bring your right leg up and place your ankle or lower leg just above your left knee, with your right leg turned out and the knee flexed at about a 90-degree angle. Keeping your right foot flexed, hinge at your hips until you feel a stretch in your right outer thigh. Repeat on the other side.

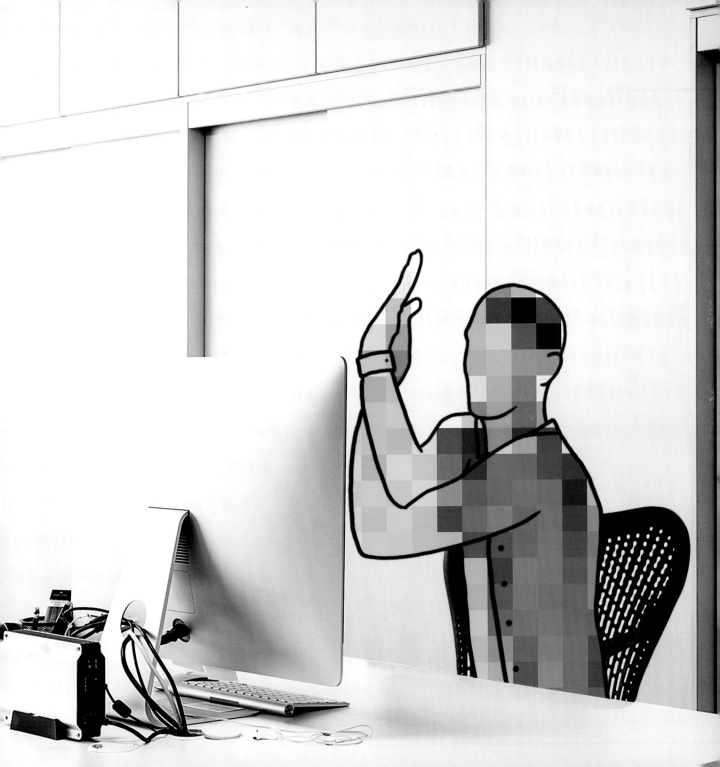

YOGA FOR EXECUTIVES

Stressed out CEOs no longer reach for a post-work martini to calm their nerves. They instead grab their yoga mat. Yoga and mindfulness practices have become ubiquitous in successful tech companies throughout Silicon Valley and even on Wall Street. Research has shown that our minds have a tendency to wander about 50 percent of the time. The daily distraction of Facebook, Instagram, email, and text messages make it harder than ever to stay focused. Meditation training has been shown to help strengthen our ability to stay focused and even boost memory. Whether you have writers block or are struggling to come up with an original new marketing strategy, a few deep breaths can help fuel your creativity. Meditation encourages divergent thinking, a key component of creativity. Research has also shown that we come up with our biggest breakthroughs and insights when we are in a relaxed state of mind. Many studies have shown that yoga decreases anxiety and can help boost performance under stress. If you're feeling anxious about a big presentation or feel constant panic day-to-day on the trading floor, try incorporating some basic breath work into your daily routine to calm your nerves.

GOPI KALLAYIL

CHIEF EVANGELIST FOR BRAND

MARKETING AT GOOGLE

Yoga has always been a big part of my life. When I joined Google, I started a group called Yoglers, a yoga program for Googlers, which is what we call those who work there. Now the program has become part of Google culture.

In our hyper-connected world, where more people have access to mobile phones than clean drinking water, we're inundated with new technology, but the most important technology we work with comes from within—our brains, our breath, our minds, our bodies, our consciousness. Yoga and meditation help us optimize this inner technology in order to allow us to live better. Daily life, especially in the workplace, is full of distractions. Yoga teaches us to distill our thoughts and actions to what is necessary in that very moment. It's easy, especially in Silicon Valley, to say you don't have time. I once set a goal of doing sixty minutes of yoga and thirty minutes of meditation every day, but work commitments got in the way. I failed. Then a good friend of mine, Chade-Meng Tan, suggested I start small, with one breath, one minute of yoga, and one minute of meditation. In each day, I can always find one minute, and so I started with this new goal and, after a week, I found that often my sessions became longer. I realized that what I was rushing off to could wait for one extra minute—or five, or more. Nothing is more important than the body and breath.

YOGA ON THE GO

Travel puts incredible stress on the body, but it's usually a go-to excuse for lapsing from a workout routine or yoga practice. Rather than seeing travel as a reason not to exercise, think of it as an opportunity to try something new: a new yoga studio, a new morning yoga sequence to help with jet lag, yoga on the beach, or even yoga on a paddleboard.

YOGA AT THE HOTEL

In the world of travel, yoga isn't just offered at fancy spa resorts. Today, many business hotels offer yoga, sometimes in dedicated studios or within the hotel gym, or via classes streamed through the TV in your room. Some even provide yoga mats in rooms and offer private sessions. Most hotel yoga classes are geared toward all levels of practice. If you're looking for a specific style of yoga or a more advanced class, ask the concierge to print out schedules of nearby yoga studios.

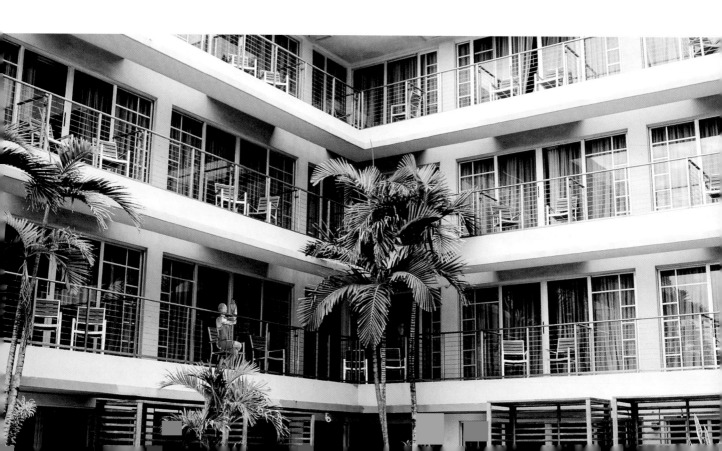

EXPERT ADVICE

(ON YOGA TO COMBAT TRAVEL FATIGUE)

When I first started touring with Maroon 5 almost a decade ago, there were only a handful of artists, like Sting and Madonna, who brought their yoga teachers with them on the road. Now everyone from Kelly Clarkson to Harry Styles seems to be doing it. Musicians are realizing the importance of maintaining a healthy body and mind on the road. Yoga is the one sutra, or thread, of consistency and stability in an ever-changing world of planes, hotels, faces, and time zones. It's indispensable to touring. The first thing Adam Levine always did, even after a sixteen-hour flight, was go right to the hotel sauna, then do ninety minutes to two hours of yoga. It's one of the best ways to reset your clock. By the time night comes, you're just exhausted and will sleep straight through until morning. Yoga is the best cure for jet lag. Once Adam had to fly to New York City just for the day to be on Saturday Night Live. He wanted to practice yoga between skits.

—CHAD DENNIS
DIRECTOR OF YOGA AT WANDERLUST HOLLYWOOD

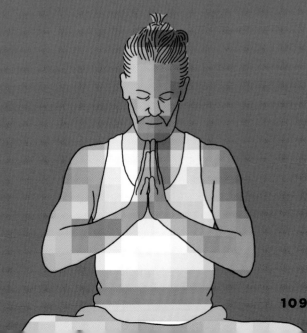

YOGA FOR THE CAR, TRAIN, OR BUS

In case you haven't heard, sitting is the new smoking—it can be just that bad for your health. If a long commute is part of your daily routine or you're taking a long road trip, counter the effects of sitting in stop-start traffic and prevent road rage with the following simple poses. If you're driving, you should obviously only perform them at red lights, gas stations, or rest stops. But if you're on a bus or train, step into the aisle and go for it!

FIVE POSES FOR THE CAR, TRAIN, OR BUS

1. If you're in traffic, a few rounds of alternate nostril breathing (page 67) can help keep road rage at bay.

2. If you've been nodding off in the passenger's seat, your neck probably paid a price. This simple stretch can undo some of the damage: Sit upright, then lean your right ear toward your right shoulder and wrap your right arm around the left side of your head, touching your left ear. Breathe deeply into your chest and the length in the left side of your neck for five breaths. Slowly roll your head to the front, bringing your chin down, and then roll it over to the left side. Repeat the stretch on the left. This also works wonders on a long flight.

3. At a rest stop, try putting your feet up on the dashboard to get blood circulating. Of course, if you're a passenger, you can do this anytime.

4. If you've got an achy butt and hips, try doing standing figure four pose at the next rest stop. Stand and place your right ankle above your left knee, turning your right leg out to create a figure four. Hinge your hips back to stretch your right hip and lower back, holding on to the car or something else for balance if need be. This will release tension from your external hip rotators and glutes.

5. At a rest stop, step back into warrior 1 (page 176) to lengthen your hip flexors and calf muscles.

EXPERT ADVICE

(ON AVOIDING BACK PAIN)

One of the most common causes of low back pain is sitting for long periods of time over many months. Your glute muscles stop firing the way they're supposed to. If you sit a lot, you need to strengthen the gluteus maximus, medius, and minimus.

For gluteus maximus strength: From table (page 172), keep your hips squared and, exhaling, draw your right knee to your nose. Then, as you inhale, slowly swing your right leg back and up so the knee is at a 90-degree angle and the bottom of the right foot is facing the ceiling. Repeat for five breaths, using slow, controlled motion, and then switch sides.

For gluteus medius strength: Side plank (page 166) is one of the best activators of the gluteus medius. Once you can comfortably hold side plank, raise the top leg to really work the abductors.

For gluteus minimus strength: One-leg balance poses, like extended hand to big toe (page 141), engage the gluteus minimus to stabilize the femur relative to the pelvis.

For all three gluteal muscles: Half-moon pose (page 147) engages all three gluteal muscles to stabilize the hip and lengthen the lower back. The gluteus maximus is used to lift the raised leg and rotate the thigh of the standing leg to open the hip; the gluteus medius stabilizes the hip of the standing leg; and the gluteus minimus allows you to bend at the hip of the standing leg and abduct the thigh of the raised leg.

—DAVID MAGONE
FOUNDER OF PRANAVAYU YOGA

YOGA ON THE PLANE

Flying is a recipe for stress and tightness. First, you're seated in a cramped, flexed position in a tiny seat for hours, which shortens the hamstrings and compresses the spine. Then there's the low pressure and low humidity, which cause swelling and dehydration. And all too often, it's an experience marked by stress and anxiety due to delays, missed connections, turbulence, or that two-year-old kicking the back of your seat on a red-eye. Throw in the germs from recycled air and jet lag, and it's no wonder that so many people get sick after a long flight. Think of yoga as a way to undo the damage of flying. Simple breathing exercises can help you stay calm or maybe even nod off. And a few easy yoga poses can help bring your body back into balance after you've been squeezed into such unnatural positions.

On long flights, try to get up at least once per hour to stretch and prevent deep vein thrombosis, a condition that occurs when a blood clot forms in one of the deep veins in the body. The goal is to move your body in the opposite direction of the flexed, seated position to bring it back into balance. Use the aisles, the back of the plane, or even the bathroom as places to stretch. There are also some simple poses you can do in your seat that probably won't bother your neighbors.

FIVE POSES FOR THE PLANE

1. Sit up straight in your seat and perform a few rounds of seated cat and cow (page 128) to stretch out your spine.

2. Reach your arms overhead, then bend deeply to the left. Return to center and then bend deeply to the right. This can be performed seated if you have enough room, or standing in the aisle.

3. Step into the aisle and do a few rounds of crescent lunge (page 135) to stretch out your hip flexors.

4. Stand on one leg and pull the heel of the other foot toward your butt to stretch your quads.

5. In a standing position, place your hands on your lower back and gently bend backward to open up your chest, upper back, and psoas.

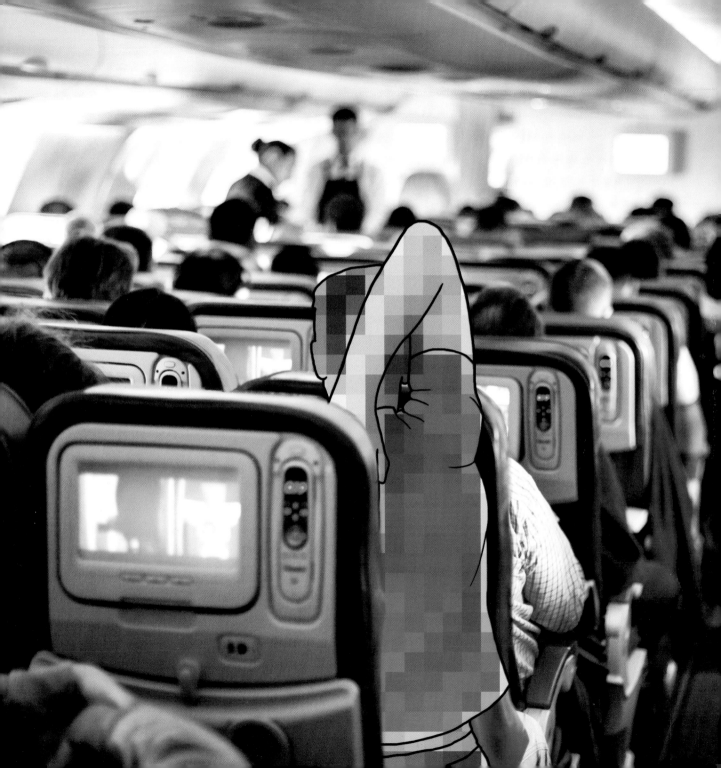

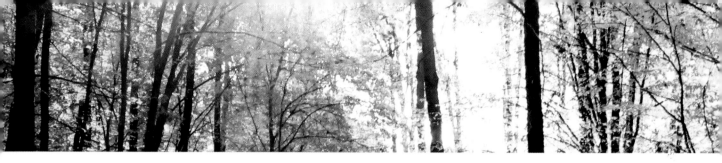

YOGA OUTDOORS

When it's a gorgeous, sunny summer day, it can be hard to motivate yourself to spend an hour confined in a yoga studio. Practicing outdoors brings its own benefits and challenges. If you're on vacation in Jackson Hole or Aspen, the mountain setting may help you relax more quickly at the start of your practice, but the altitude may make it more challenging to keep your breathing even. If you're on the beach, the sound of the ocean and wind can have a very soothing effect, but the unsteady surface of the sand and surrounding distractions can make even basic poses difficult. Be aware of the challenges of your new setting and adjust accordingly.

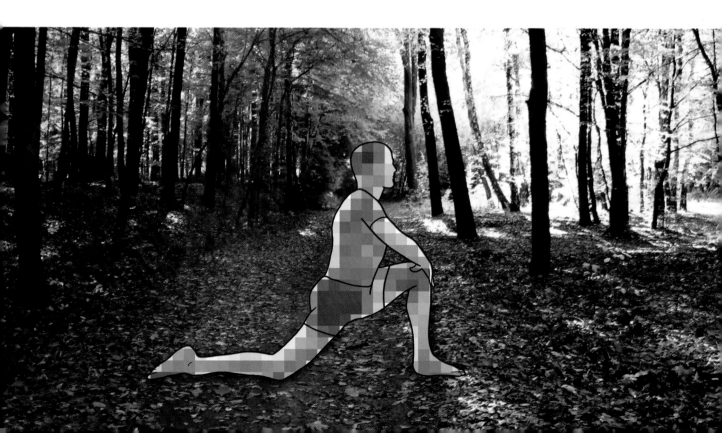

EXPERT ADVICE

(ON PRACTICING AT THE BEACH)

Yoga is about being present and sinking into the moment. When we're more relaxed, we can breathe more deeply and sink into our poses more deeply. An ocean setting helps calm the mind. Just think of how you feel when you step onto the beach on that first day of vacation. A weight drops from your shoulders. Practicing in front of the ocean, whether on the sand or from an oceanfront studio, can help clear the mind and sharpen our focus. Staring into the ocean feels like staring into infinity, and I find it much easier to fall into a trancelike state when I'm looking out to the horizon. Practicing on the beach also exposes us to the negative ions of the ocean, which have been scientifically proven to boost our mood and our immune system. The instability of the sand will make balancing postures and certain sequences challenging, but it will also engage the core and awaken small, stabilizing muscles. Poses will be slightly different in the sand. For example, in downward dog, you won't get as much mobility in the ankles to open up the calves because your toes will dig into the sand and your heels won't drop as much. I actually think sand is one of the best surfaces for beginners to start on because it's more forgiving on the knees and shins and gives inflexible people a little more comfort since they can sink down.

—CHRIS VLAUN
COFOUNDER OF V ART OF WELLNESS

YOGA AS VACATION

If the distractions of daily life have prevented you from trying yoga, why not get introduced to the practice in paradise? Vacation is about relaxation. Yoga is about relaxation. Combine the two and you'll probably be pretty blissed-out. Retreats offer an opportunity to get to know a teacher better, practice in a beautiful place with a like-minded group of people, and deepen your practice. Not all retreats have to be virtuous, ashram-like experiences. Plenty of yoga retreats now combine yoga with other activities like surfing, snowboarding, cooking, and even suspension training (think TRX). One of the best ways to find a retreat is by looking on the website of your teacher or a teacher you'd like to practice with. Remember, the location might be dreamy, but you want to be sure you're learning from a teacher whose personality and yoga style match your own. Also, look at the itinerary. Silent meditation, vegan meals, and three vinyasa sessions a day could be your idea of heaven—or hell.

A ten-day retreat at the Southwest Vipassana Meditation Center left me completely transformed. Those ten days gave me so much clarity and clarity, leads to great decisions.

KHAJAK KELEDJIAN

COFOUNDER OF THE LUXURY FASHION RETAILER INTERMIX AND FOUNDER OF INSCAPE, A MEDITATION CENTER IN NYC

THREE RETREATS TO DEEPEN YOUR PRACTICE

Kripalu Center for Yoga and Health

Where: Stockbridge, Massachusetts

What: R&R Retreats at this 160,000-square-foot wellness center let you piece together your days with options including kayaking, hiking, massage, vigorous vinyasa, qigong, and lectures on ayurveda and postural alignment. Accommodations are stark and dorm-style, though comfortable. Food is organic and vegetarian, and breakfast is taken in silence. No alcohol.

Who: Serious, curious yogis who want to invest in deepening their practice

How: *kripalu.org*

Lumeria

Where: Haiku, Maui

What: Set in Upcountry Maui, this upscale retreat offers daily classes, luxe accommodations, and farm-to-table meals (though no alcohol). Craft your own stay and combine yoga, surfing, standup paddleboarding, and hiking; or book set retreats led by yoga stars like Jason Crandell.

Who: Health-conscious foodies; surfers and wannabe surfers; beginners looking for exposure to a variety of styles

How: *lumeriamaui.com*

Yoga Farm

Where: Punta Banco, Costa Rica

What: This rustic retreat has a hippie vibe and a hillside location that overlooks the beach. Classes are held in an open-air, thatched-roof studio surrounded by jungle, and downtime allows for surfing, fishing, and hiking. You'll be vegetarian for the week and rooms are shared, though three studios are available upon request.

Who: Free spirits looking for an affordable yoga retreat by the beach; yogis who don't mind communal living or the smell of patchouli.

How: *yogafarmcostarica.org*

FIVE YOGA FESTIVALS FOR YOUR PRACTICE

Hanuman Festival

Where: Boulder, Colorado

When: June

What: Boulder is a yoga mecca, home to dozens of studios and cult teachers, including Richard Freeman and Gina Caputo. It's also home to the headquarters of *Yoga Journal.* The four-day outdoor festival attracts yoga teachers from around the globe, and free community classes are offered each day. Ticket holders get complete access to two-hour yoga classes, concerts, guided climbing, and guided hikes.

Who: A mix of crunchy granola types, yippies, hikers, and rock climbers

How: *hanumanfestival.com*

Sedona Yoga Festival

Where: Sedona, Arizona

When: March

What: Sedona is renowned as a center for spiritual energy and healing. This three-day festival features seventy-seven presenters, more than two hundred workshops, and thirty-three "conscious" vendors. Lectures and workshops focus on topics ranging from bereavement to yoga photography. Classes are complemented by hikes, energy work, and stargazing sessions.

Who: Spiritual seekers; guys looking to learn more about the therapeutic benefits of yoga; outdoor enthusiasts

How: *sedonayogafestival.com*

Shakti Fest

Where: Joshua Tree, California

When: May

What: Think of Shakti Fest as the drug-free, spiritual counterpart to Burning Man. This five-day festival celebrates the devotional paths of yoga. You'll eat organic vegetarian food, take yoga classes, and attend spiritual lectures by day, then sing and dance to *kirtan*, a sacred form of call-and-response music, under the stars late into the night.

Who: Music and dance lovers; spiritual yogis; outdoor enthusiasts

How: *shaktifest.bhaktifest.com*

Telluride Yoga Festival

Where: Telluride, Colorado

When: July

What: This is the perfect yoga festival for athletes. You can spend your mornings or afternoons mountain biking, hiking, or climbing a *via ferrata*, then treat your sore muscles to yoga sessions. Throughout the four days, lectures take place over cocktails or out on the trails, and six-hour immersion classes let you dive deep into aspects of yoga practice. In the evenings, expect to dance at DJ parties.

Who: Outdoor enthusiasts; adventurers; music lovers

How: *tellurideyogafestival.com*

Wanderlust Yoga Festivals

Where: Stratton, Vermont; Lake Tahoe, California; Oahu, Hawaii; Snowshoe, West Virginia; Whistler, British Columbia; Mont-Tremblant, Quebec; Sunshine Coast, Australia; Great Lake Taupo, New Zealand

When: Year-round

What: These four-day festivals have evolved beyond yoga to include surfing lessons, SUP yoga, slacklining, hiking, biking, farm-to-table dinners, mountaintop wine tastings, and concerts. Big-name teachers, including Rodney Yee, Eoin Finn, Elena Brower, and Janet Stone, regularly host classes.

Who: Beginner yogis looking to try new styles and mix yoga with food, music, and fun

How: *wanderlust.com/festivals*

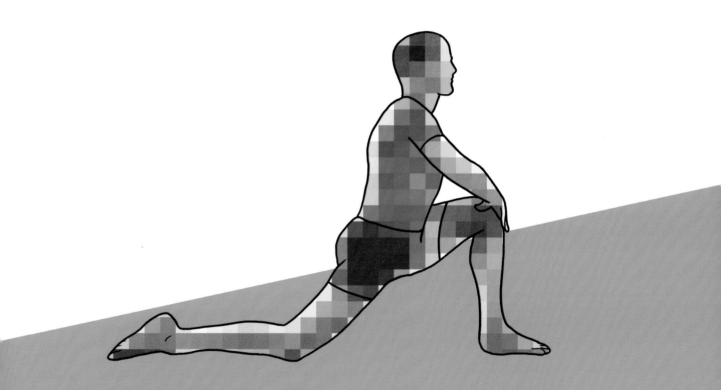

CHAPTER 7

POSES

This index of poses is not meant to be a step-by-step, how-to guide for every yoga posture. The descriptions and tips, along with the illustrations, are meant to provide a basic understanding of the various types of postures, each posture's benefits, and how to safely enter into each posture. Our index isn't a replacement for a good instructor, but it will help you build confidence as you embrace your practice and work on foundational postures at home or at a studio.

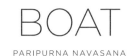

BOAT

PARIPURNA NAVASANA

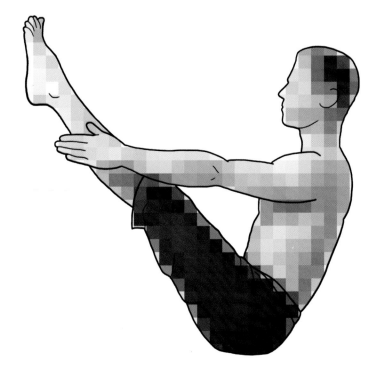

Type of pose: A seated core strengthener.

What it's good for: Strengthens the abs, hip flexors, and spine; relieves stress; improves digestion; stimulates the kidneys, intestines, prostate gland, and thyroid.

Key points: Start seated on the floor, knees bent. Place your hands behind the knees and slowly rock back and balance on your sitting bones until your toes come off the ground. Bring the knees up until the shins are parallel with the floor then slowly straighten the legs. Your body

should be in a V shape, balanced on your sitting bones. Don't let your lower back sag. Keep your chest lifted and extend your arms forward, parallel to the floor with your palms facing each other.

Modifications: Bend your knees and place your hands behind your thighs, or bend your knees and place your hands on the floor behind you. Loop a strap around the soles of your feet and push your feet against the strap as you straighten your legs and lean your torso back.

BOW

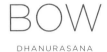

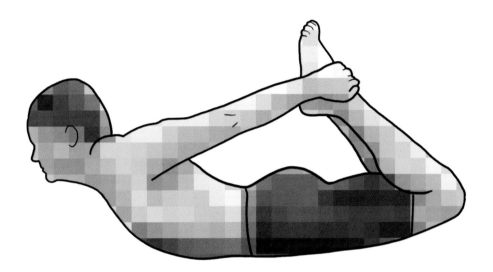

Type of pose: A heart opener and backbend.

What it's good for: Therapeutic for fatigue, constipation, anxiety, and back pain; stretches the quads and psoas; strengthens the back; stimulates the abdominal organs; improves posture; opens the chest and throat.

Key points: Bring your heels as close as you can to your butt, keeping your knees hip-distance apart, then clasp your hands around your outer ankles and lift upward. Don't let your knees splay out wider than your hips.

Modifications: If you can't hold on to your ankles, wrap a strap around the fronts of your ankles and hold the ends of the strap, keeping your arms extended. If you can't lift your thighs off the floor, place a rolled blanket beneath them for support.

BRIDGE

SETU BANDHA SARVANGASANA

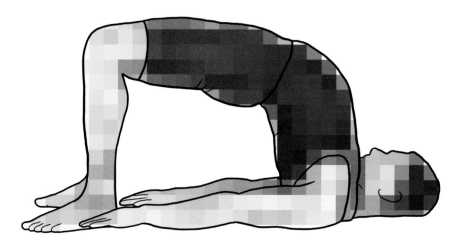

Type of pose: A backbend and mild inversion.

What it's good for: Stretches the chest and neck; opens the middle and upper back; lengthens the hip flexors; reduces anxiety, insomnia, and back pain.

Key points: Your feet should be hip-distance apart. Keep your thighs and the inside edges of your feet parallel. Your shoulders, not your neck, should be supporting the full weight of your body. If your shoulders are tight, keep your hands alongside your body with your palms pressing into the mat as you raise your hips into the air. To go deeper, draw your shoulder blades together as you extend your arms beneath your torso and clasp your hands. Keep your neck loose by lifting your chin away from your body. Avoid turning your neck from side to side.

Modifications: To prevent your legs from turning out, place a block between your feet, hip-distance apart, and keep the inner edges of your feet alongside the block as you come into the pose. Place a second block between your inner thighs to keep your knees hip-distance apart. If you feel pain in your lower back, try supporting the lift of your pelvis by placing your hands, a block, or a bolster under your sacrum for support while still keeping your legs active. If you're a beginner, you may want to place a folded blanket or towel under your shoulders to protect your neck.

Next level: Once you've mastered the pose, extend one leg straight up in the air while keeping your hips level.

BUTTERFLY, OR BOUND ANGLE

BADDHA KONASANA

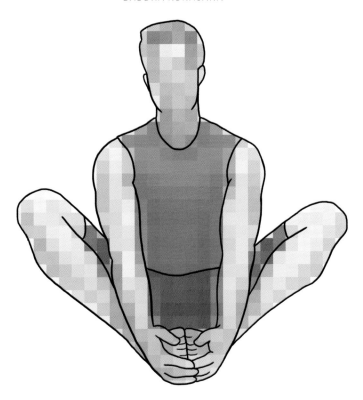

Type of pose: A seated forward fold and hip opener.

What it's good for: Stimulates the abdominal organs, kidneys, bladder, prostate gland, and heart; improves circulation; stretches the inner thighs and groins; relieves anxiety and fatigue; therapeutic for flat feet, asthma, and high blood pressure.

Key points: Press the soles of your feet together and pull your heels toward your pelvis as you drop your knees out to the sides. Keep the outer edges of your feet on the floor. If you can't hold your toes, hold your ankles or shins. Hinge from your hips, keeping your back long. Avoid rounding your spine and shoulders.

Modifications: If your knees are high off the floor and your back is rounded, sit on a block, bolster, or blanket. You may also want to place a block or folded blanket beneath each thigh to help your hips release.

CAMEL

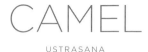

USTRASANA

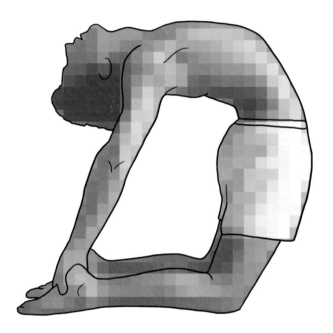

Type of pose: A heart opener and backbend.

What it's good for: Therapeutic for fatigue, anxiety, back pain, and respiratory problems; stretches the quads, groins, abdomen, chest, and psoas; strengthens the back muscles; improves posture; stimulates the abdominal organs; improves digestion.

Key points: Kneel with your knees hip-width apart, spine straight. Rotate your thighs inward and press your shins and the tops of your feet into the mat. Keep your thighs perpendicular to the floor as you slowly lean back, and try not to grip your glutes. Rest your hands, fingers pointed down, on your sacrum and keep your chin slightly tucked toward your chest as you bend backward. Then rest your palms on your heels and allow your head to drop back without crunching your neck.

Modifications: If you can't touch your hands to your heels, tuck your toes under your feet to raise them; alternatively, place a block just outside of each heel and rest your hands on the blocks.

CAT

MARJARYASANA

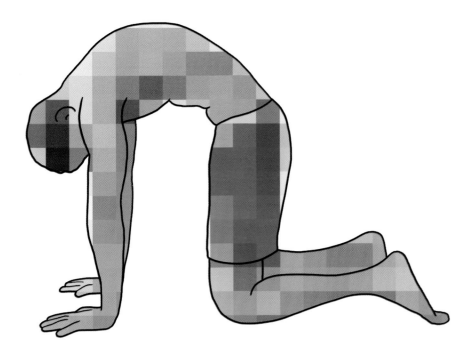

Type of pose: A core strengthener.

What it's good for: Stretches the back, torso, and neck.

Key points: Make sure that your knees are directly below your hips and that your wrists, elbows, and shoulders are aligned vertically, perpendicular to the floor. Allow your head to drop, releasing the back of your neck. Draw your navel to your spine as you exhale.

Modifications: If you have sensitive wrists or knees, use a blanket for extra cushioning.

CAT AND COW

MARJARYASANA-BITILASANA

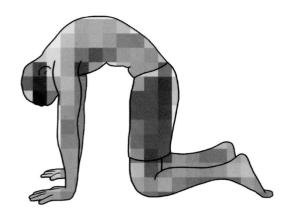 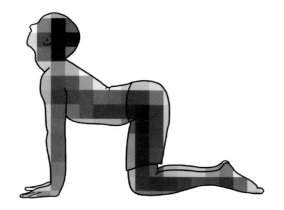

Type of pose: A gentle flow between cat (page 127), a core strengthener, and cow (page 133), a heart opener and backbend.

What it's good for: Increases flexibility in the spine; stimulates the kidneys and adrenal glands; stretches the neck, back, and front of the torso; opens the chest.

Key points: On an inhalation, gently arch your back and open your chest in cow. As you exhale, draw your naval to your spine and round your back into cat letting your head drop and releasing the back of your neck.

Modifications: If you have neck or wrist pain, you can practice this pose in a seated position. Start in easy pose (page 140) and place the tops of your hands gently on your knees. On an inhale, gently arch your back and open your chest. As you exhale, draw your naval to your spine and round your back, letting your head drop and releasing the back of your neck. If you work at a desk, you can practice this pose throughout your day. Sitting in a chair with your feet flat on the floor, press your hands against a desk or wall in front of you and perform the same spinal movements as above.

CHAIR

UTKATASANA

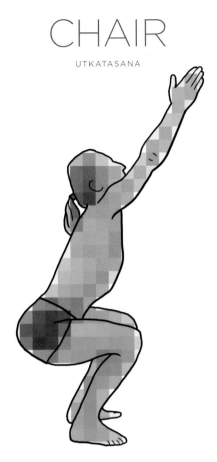

Type of pose: A standing core strengthener.

What it's good for: Stimulates the abdominal organs, diaphragm, circulatory system, and heart; stretches the shoulders and chest; strengthens the ankles, thighs, calves, and spine; therapeutic for flat feet.

Key points: Start with your feet hip-width apart and eventually work toward having your feet together, big toes touching. As you sink your hips back, keep your weight in your heels to the point that you could lift your toes off the mat. Maintain a slight arch in your back as you draw your chest back and up.

Modifications: Strengthen your abductors by squeezing a block between your inner thighs.

Next level: Once in chair pose, challenge your balance by lifting up onto the balls of your feet.

CHILD'S POSE

BALASANA

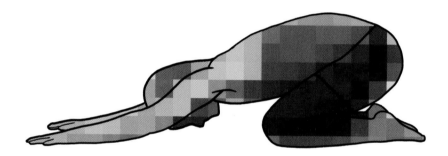

Type of pose: A restorative forward fold and hip opener.

What it's good for: Stretches the thighs, hips, and ankles; relives back pain; calms the mind; relieves stress and fatigue; used as a resting pose between more difficult postures.

Key points: Your knees should be spread apart, and your big toes should be touching. Rest your chest and forehead, and extend your arms toward the front of the mat, palms facing down.

Modifications: If you have tight hips, keep your knees and thighs together (sometimes called embryo pose). Rest your chest on top of your thighs and your forehead on the mat. Bring your arms alongside your thighs, palms up.

COBRA

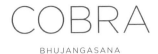

BHUJANGASANA

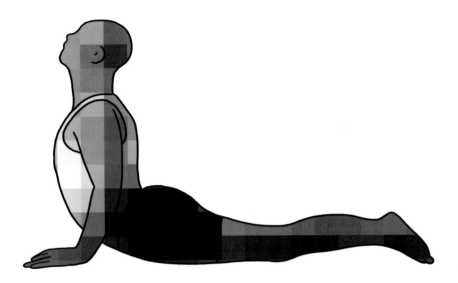

Type of pose: A heart opener and backbend.

What it's good for: Counteracts the slouch that comes from sitting in front of a computer; increases flexibility in the spine; stretches the chest, shoulders, and abdomen; opens the heart and lungs; relieves stress and fatigue; soothes sciatica.

Key points: Your hands should be beneath your shoulders when you begin. As you straighten your arms to lift your chest off the floor, hug your elbows into your body. The more you engage your legs by pressing them firmly on the floor, the easier it will be to lift your chest higher in the pose. Keep your shoulders dropped away from your ears so you don't crunch your neck. There should be very little weight in your hands; the lift comes from the strength of the spine. Don't overdo the backbend.

Modifications: If your shoulders are stiff or you simply aren't in a place where you can lie down, stand facing a wall and place your palms against the wall with your elbows hugged in to your sides. As you press against the wall, draw your shoulder blades into your upper back and broaden across your collarbones.

Next level: Deepen the challenge by lifting your palms off the floor while keeping your chest lifted. Advance to upward dog (page 174).

CORPSE

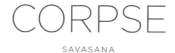

SAVASANA

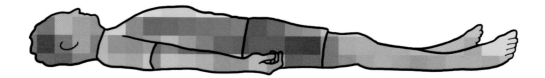

Type of pose: A restorative pose.

What it's good for: Reduces headaches and insomnia; helps lower blood pressure; lowers heart rate; calms the mind and relaxes the body; relieves stress and fatigue.

Key points: Breathe naturally and let your feet drop open. The body often cools down in *savasana*, so cover yourself with a blanket or keep a sweatshirt and socks nearby. And remember, this isn't time to sleep; though it may be challenging, the aim is to be present and aware while fully relaxed.

Modifications: If your lower back is tight, place a bolster or rolled blanket under your knees to allow your lower back to relax.

COW

BITILASANA

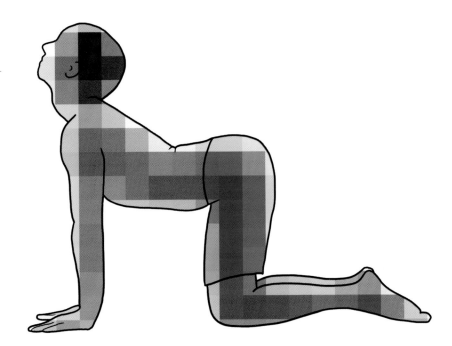

Type of pose: A heart opener and backbend.

What it's good for: Stretches the neck and the front of the torso.

Key points: Make sure that your knees are directly below your hips and that your wrists, elbows, and shoulders are aligned vertically, perpendicular to the floor. The movement should start with raising your tailbone as you inhale; gently extending your neck and head should be the last part of the movement. Protect your neck by drawing your shoulders down, away from your ears.

Modifications: If you have sensitive wrists or knees, use a blanket for extra cushioning.

Next level: Combine as a flowing sequence with cat pose (page 127) to warm up your spine.

COW FACE

GOMUKHASANA

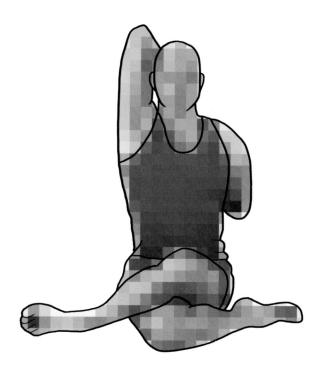 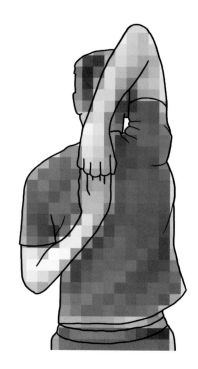

Type of pose: A seated hip and heart opener.

What it's good for: Stretches the hips, shoulders, ankles, thighs, triceps, and chest; improves postural alignment; calms the mind; reduces stress and fatigue; increases blood supply to the legs and arms.

Key points: You want to have one knee stacked directly above the other, with your sitting bones firmly on the floor. Don't let your elbows extend out to the sides; draw them in toward your body. Your top elbow should reach toward the ceiling while your lower elbow reaches toward the floor.

Modifications: If both sitting bones aren't firmly on the ground, sit on a blanket or bolster. If you have tight shoulders and can't clasp your hands behind your back, use a strap or a twisted T-shirt.

CRESCENT LUNGE, OR LOW LUNGE

ANJANEYASANA

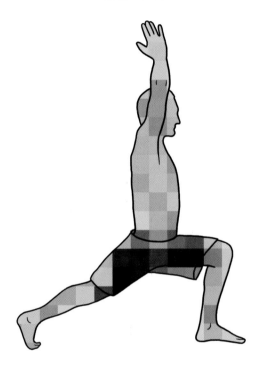

Type of pose: A standing balance pose and heart opener.

What it's good for: Stretches the groins, hip flexors, and legs; opens the chest, shoulders, and front of the torso; strengthens the thighs and glutes; improves balance; increases energy.

Key points: Make sure your front knee stays aligned with your front ankle, with your front shin perpendicular to the floor. Keep your feet hip-width apart. Draw the hip of your front leg back and the other hip forward. Spin your pinky fingers toward each other, opening your arms so your palms face each other as you raise them. Keep your tailbone tucked under and your abs engaged.

Modifications: If you feel unsteady, lower your back knee to the floor.

Next level: Advance to revolved crescent lunge (page 162).

CROW

BAKASANA

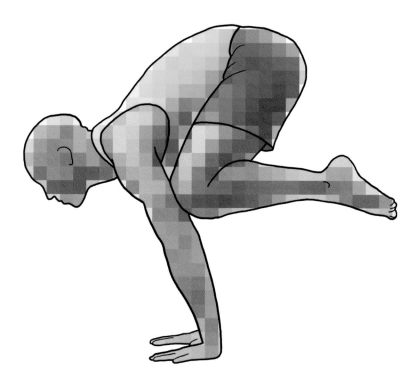

Type of pose: An arm balance and core strengthener.

What it's good for: Stretches the upper back, arms, wrists, and groins; strengthens the abdominal muscles; improves balance.

Key points: From wide squat (page 181), lower your palms to the floor, rise onto your toes, and tip forward bringing your knees behind your elbows. Tuck in tightly, keeping your heels close to your butt. Keep your gaze forward without compressing your neck. Don't let your elbows splay out to the sides, and keep your weight in your fingertips rather than your wrists.

Modifications: If you initially have difficulty getting into the pose, try lifting one leg at a time. Alternatively, try placing blocks under your feet and squatting on them so your feet are a few inches off the floor, which makes it easier to come into the pose.

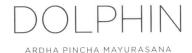

DOLPHIN

ARDHA PINCHA MAYURASANA

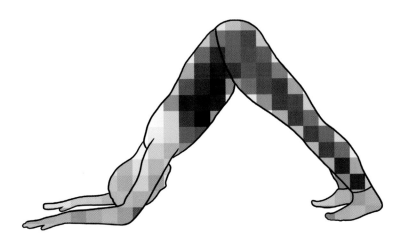

Type of pose: A standing core strengthener and mild inversion.

What it's good for: Relieves stress; strengthens the arms and legs; stretches the shoulders and hamstrings; improves digestion; therapeutic for high blood pressure and sciatica; calms the mind.

Key points: From table (page 172) place your forearms on the floor with your shoulders directly above your wrists. Keep your forearms parallel to each other as you press your forearms and palms into the floor. Tuck your toes and lift your knees off the floor, keeping them bent

as you lengthen your spine. Slowly straighten your legs until your torso and legs form an A shape. Align your ears with your upper arms and keep your head relaxed, gazing between your legs. Your heels need not touch the floor.

Modifications: If your upper back rounds when you try to straighten your legs, keep them bent until you gain flexibility in your spine. Clasp your hands together to help open your shoulders.

Next level: To build core strength, lower yourself into forearm plank (page 144), then press back into dolphin. Repeat a few times.

DOWNWARD DOG

ADHO MUKHA SVANASANA

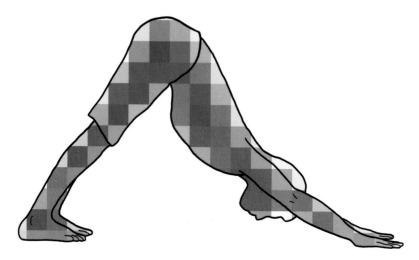

Type of pose: A foundational and transitional pose and mild inversion.

What it's good for: Calms the mind; increases energy; stretches the shoulders, hands, hamstrings, calves, and arches of the feet; strengthens the arms, shoulders, and legs; relieves fatigue, insomnia, and stress; therapeutic for sciatica, flat feet, and high blood pressure.

Key points: The folds of your wrists should be parallel to the top edge of your mat, and your middle fingers should point directly to the top edge of your mat. Distribute your weight evenly across your hands, pressing firmly through your palms and knuckles and actively pressing the bases of your index fingers into the floor. Firm your outer arms and, as you push your hips up, firm your shoulder blades against your back, then widen them and draw them toward your tailbone. Keep your head between your upper arms, not hanging down or looking up. Don't worry about your heels touching the ground, and don't lock your knees; it's okay to keep them slightly bent for comfort. Your back should be flat, not rounded.

Modifications: If you have tight shoulders, you can try placing your hands on blocks. To get in the habit of engaging your arms, loop a strap just above your elbows and push your inner shoulder blades outward as you resist the strap. Grip a block between your inner thighs and press it toward the wall behind you to promote inner rotation of your thighs. If you have wrist pain, drop your forearms to dolphin (page 137).

Next level: Keeping your hips level, raise one leg and hold it in alignment with your torso.

EAGLE

GARUDASANA

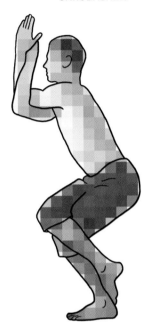

Type of pose: A standing balance pose and hip opener.

What it's good for: Improves balance; strengthens and stretches the ankles and calves; stretches the thighs, hips, shoulders, and upper back; opens the back of the lungs; therapeutic for low back pain and asthma.

Key points: Start in chair (page 129). Put your weight in your left leg as you lift and cross your right leg over your left thigh. Hook the top of your right foot over your left calf. Extend your arms straight out in front of you and drop your right arm under your left. Bend your elbows, then raise your forearms perpendicular to the floor. Wrap your arms and hands and try to get your palms as close to touching as possible. Squeezing your thighs and arms together will help with balance. Your elbows should stay lifted as your shoulder blades press down your back.

Modifications: If you have trouble hooking the foot of your raised leg behind the calf of your standing leg, press the big toe of the raised foot against the floor instead, for extra balance. If your palms don't touch in the wrap, press the backs of your hands together or hold a strap and keep it taut between your hands as you wrap your arms.

EASY POSE

SUKHASANA

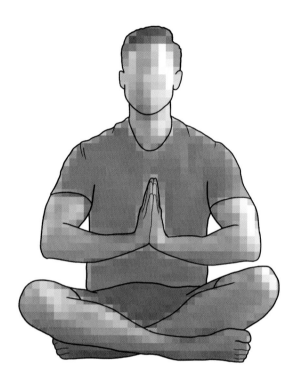

Type of pose: A foundational seated pose and hip opener.

What it's good for: Calms the mind; strengthens the back; stretches hips, groins, and outer thighs.

Key points: Balance on both sitting bones. Relax your feet, with the outer edges resting on the floor and the inner arches resting just below the opposite shins. Place your hands on your thighs, palms facing either down or up, or bring your palms together in front of your heart in prayer position.

Modifications: If your hips are tight, sit on a blanket, bolster, or block so your hips are above the level of your knees. For more back support, you can sit with your back against a wall.

EXTENDED HAND TO BIG TOE

UTTHITA HASTA PADANGUSTASANA

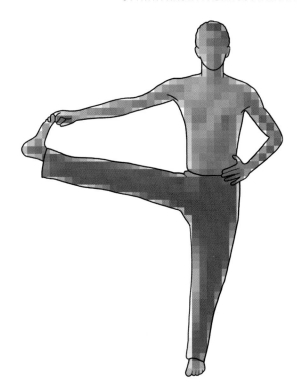

Type of pose: A standing balance pose.

What it's good for: Improves balance and focus; strengthens the legs.

Key points: Start in mountain pose (page 154). Bring your right knee to your chest. Reach your right arm inside of your right thigh and loop your index and middle fingers around your big toe. On an inhalation, extend your right leg forward, straightening the knee as much as possible. Put your left hand on your hip for balance. Keep your spine straight and your left leg engaged without locking your knee. If you are stable in the pose, extend your leg to the side.

Modifications: If you can't reach your toes start by hugging the knee of the raised leg into your chest or loop a strap around the ball of the foot.

Next level: Try holding up your extended leg without using your hand.

EXTENDED SIDE ANGLE

UTTHITA PARSVAKONASANA

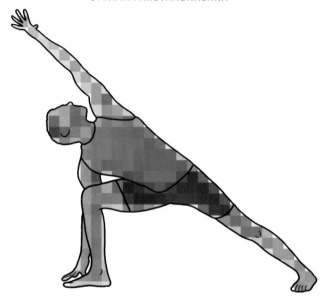

Type of pose: A standing and strengthening pose.

What it's good for: Strengthens the legs; stretches the spine, groins, chest, abdomen, and shoulders; therapeutic for constipation, sciatica, and low back pain.

Key points: From warrior 2 (page 177), lower the arm on the same side as the front leg to your thigh or the floor. Stretch the other arm up and forward, extending it over your head so your biceps is over your ear and your fingertips are reaching in the same direction as your front toes. Make sure your front knee doesn't drift inward. Keep your front thigh in external rotation by drawing your knee toward the pinky toe of your front foot.

Modifications: If you have trouble keeping your back heel flat on the floor as you bend your front knee, press it against a wall. If you struggle to touch your hand to the ground, rest your forearm on top of the thigh of your front leg, or put a block just outside your front foot and place your hand on the block.

Next level: For a deeper pose, place your front hand on the floor just outside of your front foot. To open your chest even further, go into bound extended side angle (*baddha utthita parsvakonasana*) by wrapping your bottom arm beneath the hamstring of your bent leg (from front to back) and bringing your top arm behind you to meet it until you can clasp your hands together.

EXTENDED TRIANGLE

UTTHITA TRIKONASANA

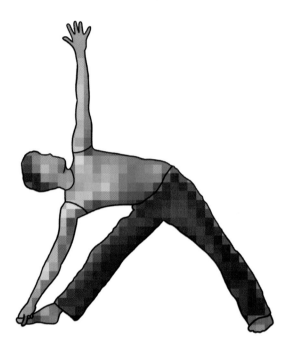

Type of pose: A standing heart opener and strengthening pose.

What it's good for: Reduces stress; improves balance; stretches the hamstrings, groins, and hips; opens the chest and shoulders; improves digestion and metabolism.

Key points: From warrior 2 (page 177), straighten the front knee. Extend your front hand forward so your chest hovers nearly parallel to the floor. Lower your front hand. If it doesn't touch the ground, place it on your thigh, your shin, or a block; don't rest it directly on your knee. Keep your head in a neutral position or softly gaze upward toward your top hand. Keep your front leg straight but with a microbend in the knee. Your torso should be in the same plane as your front thigh at all times. Your back leg should remain engaged, with the foot pressing firmly into the ground.

Modifications: If you feel unsteady in the pose, press your back heel against a wall or press your back into the wall.

Next level: Instead of reaching your top arm straight towards the ceiling, stretch it over the top ear, parallel to the floor.

FOREARM PLANK, OR DOLPHIN PLANK

MAKARA ADHO MUKHA SVANASANA

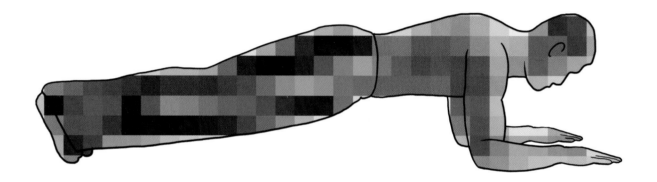

Type of pose: An arm balance and core strengthener.

What it's good for: Strengthens the arms, legs, and core; improves posture; calms the mind; improves focus.

Key points: From table (page 172), lower your elbows directly beneath your shoulders and place your forearms on the mat parallel to each other. Step your feet back, until your body forms a straight line, with your heels over your toes. Don't let your hips sink or your butt stick up in the air. Gaze between your hands.

Modifications: If your core isn't strong enough to hold the pose, lower your knees to the floor while keeping your head and spine in a straight line.

Next leve:: To build core strength, press yourself directly back into dolphin (page 137), then come back into forearm plank. Repeat a few times.

FOUR-LIMBED STAFF

CHATURANGA DANDASANA

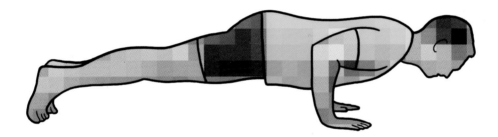

Type of pose: An arm balance and core strengthener and transitional pose.

What it's good for: Strengthens the arms, wrists, and core; improves posture.

Key points: Your body should be in one straight line, with your elbows bent at a 90-degree angle above your wrists. Don't let your shoulders drop below your elbows. Keep your elbows hugged in, toward your rib cage, and extend out through your heels.

Modifications: If your elbows splay out, loop a strap around your upper arms, just above your elbows, for support. Even advanced yogis will lose form after their thirtieth *chaturanga*. Modify by going to knees, chest, and chin pose (*ashtanga namaskara*): Lower your knees to the floor and keep your toes tucked under. Keep your hips lifted and palms flat below your elbows as you lower your chest to the floor between your hands. Lower your chin to touch the floor.

Next level: Try one-legged *chaturanga*, raising one foot to hip level or just above hip level.

HALF FRONT SPLITS

ARDHA HANUMANASANA

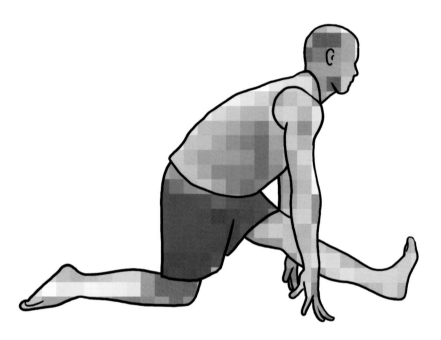

Type of pose: A hip opener.

What it's good for: Stretches the hamstrings, groins, and calf muscles.

Key points: From crescent lunge (page 135), slowly straighten out your front leg while keeping your back knee directly under your hip (in other words, don't sit your butt down on your back heel). Then flex your front foot so the heel extends forward and fold as close to the front leg as possible while drawing your abdomen in.

Modifications: If it's difficult to keep your hands steady on the ground as your front leg straightens, place a block under each hand or keep a gentle bend in your front leg. For an IT band stretch, spin the pinky toe edge of your front foot down so the outer edge of your foot is in contact with the mat. Walk your hands (or blocks if necessary) to the outside of the extended leg. Draw the hip of the front leg back without actually moving your front foot and gaze over the shoulder on the same side as the front foot.

HALF-MOON

ARDHA CHANDRASANA

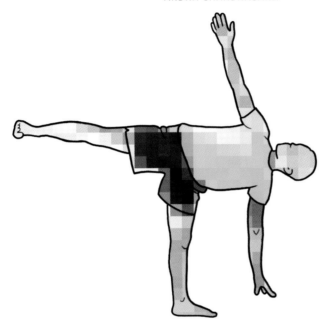

Type of pose: A standing balance strengthening pose, and mild inversion.

What it's good for: Lengthens the spine; opens the chest and shoulders; relieves stress and fatigue; improves digestion; improves balance and focus; increases proprioception.

Key points: Enter this pose from extended triangle (page 143). As you inhale, bend your front knee and slide your back foot about six inches forward along the mat. At the same time, slide your front hand forward about twelve inches beyond your front foot. Pressing your front hand into the floor, straighten the standing leg as you simultaneously lift the back leg parallel to the floor, pushing out through the heel. Rotate your torso up while keeping your gaze forward and your head in a neutral position. The top hand can be on the hip or raised straight up in line with the bottom arm.

Modifications: If it's hard to reach the floor, place a block beneath your bottom hand. If balancing is difficult, perform this pose with your back against a wall.

Next level: Bend the knee of the raised leg and grab the foot or ankle with the top hand for a quad stretch and chest opener.

HANDSTAND

ADHO MUKHA VRKSASANA

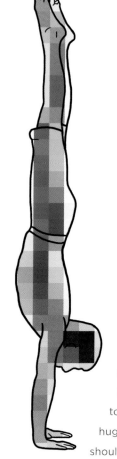

Type of pose: Balance and strengthening pose.

What it's good for: Improves balance; calms the mind; relieves stress; strengthens the shoulders, wrists, and arms.

Key points: From downward dog (page 138), walk your feet in closer to your hands. Bend one knee and keep the other leg active by extending through the heel. As you hop off the bent leg, bring the extending leg up and above your body and then bring the other leg up to meet it. Rotate your upper arms outward to keep your shoulder blades broad, while also hugging your outer arms inward. Keep your wrists, shoulders, and arms stacked, and keep the weight in your palms and fingers, rather than your wrists.

Modifications: Practice the pose against a wall. Start by taking small hops off of one leg and slowly bringing the opposite leg above the hips to balance in the air.

HAPPY BABY

ANANDA BALASANA

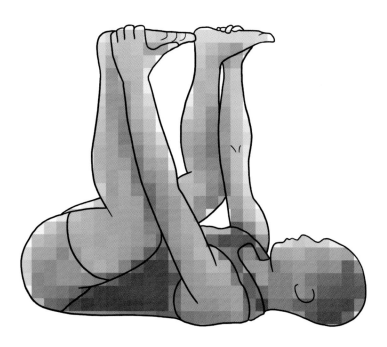

Type of pose: A hip opener.

What it's good for: Stretches the groins and back; relieves stress and fatigue; calms the mind.

Key points: Position each ankle directly over the knee, so your shins are perpendicular to the floor. Your knees should be slightly wider than your torso and should come up toward your armpits. Flex through your heels and press your tailbone into the floor.

Modifications: If your tailbone or neck comes off the mat as you reach for your feet, it means your hips are tight. In that case, you can try to grip your ankles or shins instead of your feet. Alternatively, hold on to a strap looped over the soles of your feet.

HERO

VIRASANA

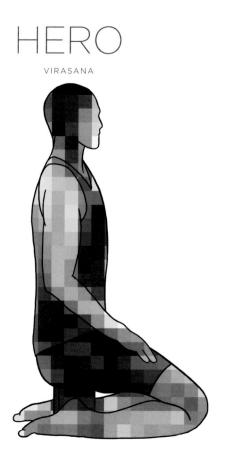

Type of pose: Seated pose.

What it's good for: Improves posture; increases flexibility in the thighs, knees, and ankles; strengthens the arches of the feet; improves digestion.

Key points: Kneel on the floor with your inner knees touching. Open your feet slightly wider than your hips and, on an exhale, slowly sink your buttocks to the floor, making sure that both sitting bones are grounded. Your heals and shins should be alongside your hips and the tops of your feet flat on the floor with the big toes angled in toward each other. Place your hands on your thighs, palms down, and sit up straight. Hold for five breaths.

Modifications: If you have knee issues, you may find it challenging to sit on the floor. Instead, sit on a block (or two) placed between your shins.

LEGS UP THE WALL

VIPARITA KARANI

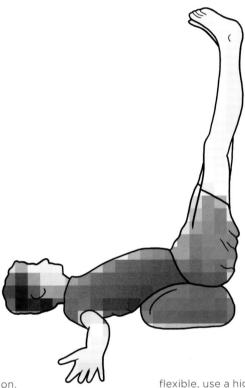

Type of pose: A restorative inversion.

What it's good for: Reduces edema in the legs and feet; calms the mind and nervous system; improves digestion; regulates blood pressure; helps with insomnia.

Key points: Use props—either a bolster or thickly folded blanket—to get the most out of this pose. If you're stiff, place your support farther from the wall. If you're more flexible, use a higher support and place it closer to the wall. Your sitting bones should drape down into the space between the support and the wall, your sternum should lift toward your chin, and your arms should be out to the sides, palms up.

Modifications: Looping a strap around your thighs, just above your knees, allows you to further relax your legs and release your inner thighs.

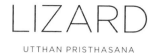

LIZARD

UTTHAN PRISTHASANA

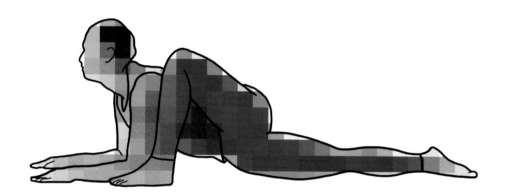

Type of pose: A hip and heart opener.

What it's good for: Stretches the psoas, groins, hamstrings, and quads; opens the chest and shoulders.

Key points: From crescent lunge (page 135), place both hands on the floor to the inside of one foot. Turn your front foot out at a 45-degree angle and roll onto the outside edge of the foot. As you bring your forearms to the ground, sink your hips forward with your back toes rooted in the mat. Keep your spine long as you sink your

chest forward. Gaze forward to keep your chest open.

Modifications: If you have tight hips, place a block under your forearms or drop the back knee.

Next level: Use the hand on the same side as your front leg to push against the inner thigh of the front leg to open up the hip. Hold for a few breaths. Then bend your back knee and catch your pinky toe edge of the back foot with the opposite hand. Pull gently to stretch the quad muscle.

LOCUST

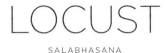

SALABHASANA

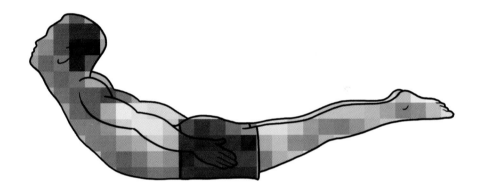

Type of pose: A chest opener and backbend.

What it's good for: Relieves indigestion, constipation, and gas; relieves stress and fatigue; stretches the shoulders, chest, and quads; strengthens the spine and glutes; stimulates the abdominal organs.

Key points: Start by lying face down. Lift your chest and arms on an exhalation. Use your inner thighs to lift your legs, rotating them inward by turning the big toes toward each other to avoid compressing your lower back. Your weight should rest on your lower ribs, stomach, and pelvis.

Modifications: Place a rolled blanket beneath your sternum to help maintain the lift in your torso. Lift one leg off the floor until you have the strength to lift both.

Next level: For a deeper shoulder stretch, interlace your fingers behind your back and reach your knuckles toward your heels.

MOUNTAIN POSE

TADASANA

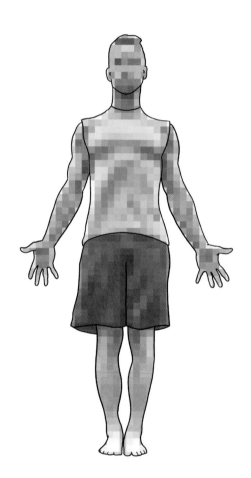

Type of pose: A foundational standing pose.

What it's good for: Improves posture; strengthens the ankles and thighs; relieves sciatica.

Key points: Stand with your big toes touching and heels slightly apart. Keep your thighs firm with your kneecaps lifted. Extend your arms by your sides. Press your shoulders back without jutting out your lower front ribs.

Modifications: If you are have trouble balancing, stand with your feet slightly farther apart.

PIGEON

EKA PADA RAJAKAPOTASANA

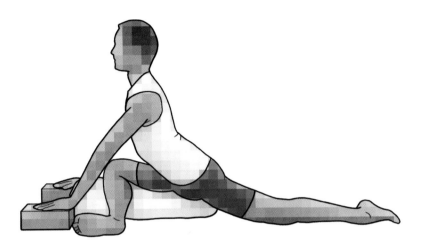

Type of pose: A hip opener.

What it's good for: Lengthens the hip flexors; stretches the glutes; improves digestion; relieves stress and fatigue; calms the mind.

Key points: From table (page 172), bring your left knee forward and place it in on the floor just behind and slightly left of your left wrist. Your shin should be on a diagonal with your left heel pointing toward your right hip. Keep your hips square to the front of the mat and your front knee in line with your hip and keep your front foot flexed to protect the knee. Work toward bringing your front shin as parallel to the front edge of your mat as possible. If you have tight hips, your front shin might remain angled back until you gain flexibility. Your back leg should extend straight out from the hip and slightly rotate inward. Try to press all fives toes of the back foot into the mat.

Modifications: If your hips are tight and the hip of your front leg comes off the floor, place a blanket or block under the sitting bone and thigh of the bent leg for support. For a restorative variation, drape your torso over your front shin and reach forward, resting your forehead on the mat.

Next level: Grab the ankle of your back foot and bend your knee for a quad stretch. In the full pose, your spine is extended in a backbend, and the toes of your back foot touch your head.

PLANK

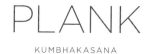

KUMBHAKASANA

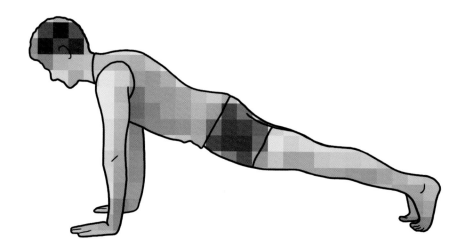

Type of pose: An arm balance and core strengthener.

What it's good for: Strengthens the arms, wrists, spine, and core; improves posture.

Key points: Your wrists should remain directly under your shoulders, with a microbend in your elbows, and your body should be in one line with your head neutral, as a natural extension of your spine. Press your quadriceps up toward the ceiling while lengthening your tailbone toward your heels.

Modifications: There's no shame in bringing your knees to the mat, especially toward the end of a class if you feel your hips sinking and arms shaking as you try to hold the pose. If you suffer from carpal tunnel syndrome or experience soreness in your wrists, come down onto your forearms for forearm plank (page 144).

Next level: Raise one of your legs parallel to the floor while keeping your hips even. Or advance to side plank (page 166).

PLOW

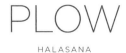

HALASANA

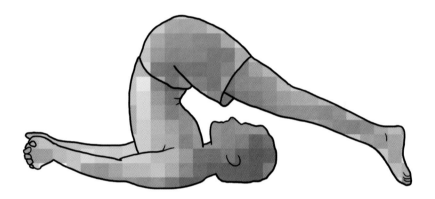

Type of pose: An inversion.

What it's good for: Improves digestion; stimulates the thyroid; stretches the neck, shoulders, and back; therapeutic for headaches and insomnia; relieves stress and fatigue.

Key points: From supported shoulder stand (page 171), slowly hinge at the hips to lower your toes to the floor behind your head. Once your feet are resting on the floor, extend your arms out on the floor in the opposite direction and press your upper arms firmly into the floor; you can clasp your hands together if you like. Keep some space between your chin and chest.

Modifications: To protect your neck, place a folded blanket beneath your shoulders. If your toes don't touch the floor, place your hands on your lower back for support and rest your feet on a bolster.

RECLINING BUTTERFLY, OR RECLINING BOUND ANGLE

SUPTA BADDHA KONASANA

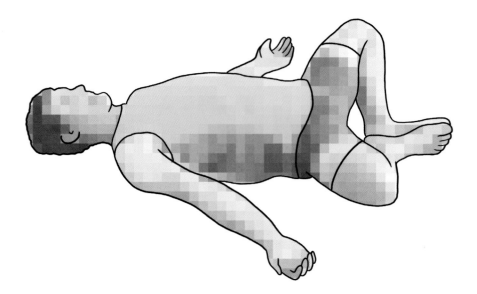

Type of pose: A restorative hip opener.

What it's good for: Lowers blood pressure; decreases heart rate; relieves fatigue and insomnia; reduces stress and muscle tension; stretches the hips, groins, and inner thigh muscles.

Key points: From butterfly (page 125), bring your elbows to the floor, then slowly lower your back to the ground.

Let your arms relax by your sides, palms facing up. Lengthen your tailbone toward your heels and relax your glute muscles.

Modifications: If you have tight hips, you may want to place a block under each knee for support. To relax more deeply into the pose, recline back onto a bolster running lengthwise beneath your spine.

RECLINING SPINAL TWIST

SUPTA MATSYENDRASANA

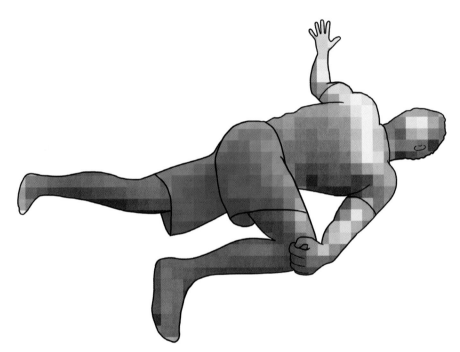

Type of pose: A restorative twist.

What it's good for: Promotes detoxification; improves digestion; reduces stress; stretches the glutes and back muscles; realigns the spine.

Key points: Lie on your back and, on an exhalation, draw your right knee to your chest keeping your left leg extended. Extend your right arm out along the floor at shoulder height. Place your left hand on the outside of your right knee and shift your hips slightly to the right. On an exhalation, lower your right knee over the left side of your body. Turn your head to gaze to the right. Try to keep both shoulder blades pressing into the floor.

Modifications: If you have tight hips, rest your top knee on a bolster.

REVERSE WARRIOR

VIPARITA VIRABHADRASANAT

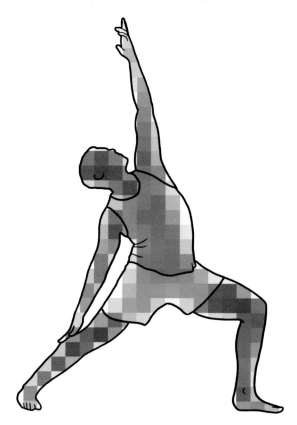

Type of pose: A standing and strengthening pose and a heart opener.

What it's good for: Strengthens and stretches the legs, groins, and sides of the body; increases flexibility in the spine; opens the chest; reduces fatigue; calms the mind.

Key points: From warrior 2 (page 177), raise your front arm up toward the ceiling as you slowly extend your spine into a gentle backbend. Keep your front knee aligned with your front ankle. Don't collapse into your lower back, and don't crunch your neck. Your back hand should rest lightly on your back leg.

Modifications: If you feel strain in your lower back, try keeping your hands on your hips as you lift your chest and lengthen your spine.

REVOLVED CHAIR

PARIVRTTA UTKATASANA

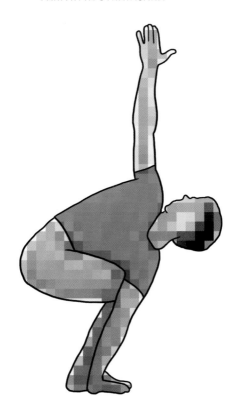

Type of pose: A standing twist and core strengthener.

What it's good for: Promotes detoxification; improves digestion; increases flexibility in the spine; improves balance; strengthens the thighs.

Key points: From chair (page 129), place your hands at your heart in prayer position and, as you inhale, twist your torso, hooking your bottom elbow onto the outer edge of your knee. Twist more deeply with every exhalation. Make sure your knees stay aligned.

Modifications: If you have trouble balancing, try taking a wider stance.

Next level: To deepen the pose, extend both arms, reaching your top fingertips to the sky and bottom fingertips to the ground.

REVOLVED CRESCENT LUNGE

PARIVRTTA ANJANEYASANA

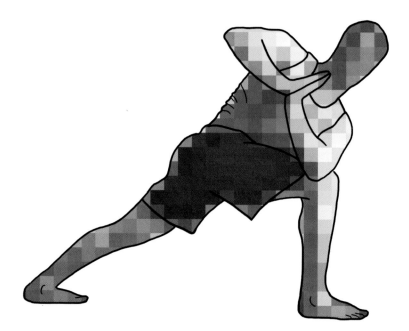

Type of pose: A standing twist and leg strengthener.

What it's good for: Strengthens the legs; opens the chest, shoulders, and torso; improves balance.

Key points: In crescent lunge (page 135), bring your palms together in prayer position at your chest and, on an exhalation, twist your torso to bring the elbow of the opposite arm to the outside of your front thigh. Press your upper arm against your thigh and draw your shoulder

blades into your back to open your chest. Twist more deeply with every exhalation. Press out through your back heel and keep the back leg engaged.

Modifications: Lower the back knee.

Next level: Extend both arms and reach the fingertips of your top arm to the sky and the fingertips of your bottom arm to the floor.

REVOLVED TRIANGLE

PARIVTTA TRIKONASANA

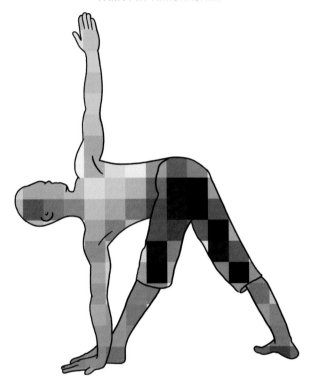

Type of pose: A standing and strengthening twist.

What it's good for: Promotoes detoxification; stretches the hamstrings and hips; opens the chest and shoulders; improves balance and focus; improves digestion; relieves stress; therapeutic for low back pain.

Key points: From mountain pose (page 154) step, your left foot back about three feet and align your heels. The front toes should point toward the top of the mat. Pivot the back foot outward to a 45-degree angle. Square your hips forward. Extend both arms out to the sides, parallel to the floor. As you exhale, hinge forward from your hips and bring your left hand to the outside of your right foot as you twist open your torso to the right. Draw your right hip back to keep it in line with your left hip. Bring your gaze to your raised hand.

Modifications: If you have trouble keeping your back heel grounded, shorten your stance or perform the pose with your back heel pressed against a wall. You can also rest your bottom hand on a block.

SEATED FORWARD FOLD

PASCHIMOTTANASANA

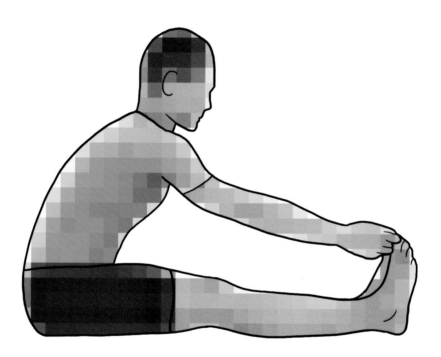

Type of pose: A seated forward fold.

What it's good for: Calms the brain and relieves stress; stimulates the liver, adrenal glands, and kidneys; stretches the spine, shoulders, and hamstrings; improves digestion; reduces fatigue; therapeutic for high blood pressure and insomnia.

Key points: This isn't about touching your toes. Hinge from the hip joints, not from the waist, and think about resting your torso on your thighs, rather than tipping your head downward to touch your knees.

Modifications: If necessary, start with your knees bent and work toward straightened legs as your flexibility increases. If you have tight hamstrings, sit on a folded blanket. If that doesn't provide sufficient relief, place a rolled blanket under your knees. You can loop a strap around the soles of your feet to help you hinge from the hips and lengthen the spine.

SEATED SPINAL TWIST, OR HALF LORD OF THE FISHES

ARDHA MATSYENDRASANA

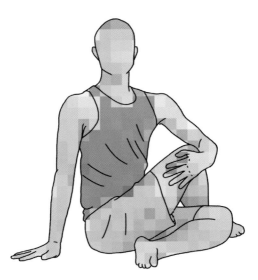

Type of pose: A seated hip opener and twist.

What it's good for: Stimulates the liver and kidneys; improves digestion and metabolism; stretches the shoulders, hips, and neck; increases flexibility of the spine; relieves fatigue and back pain.

Key points: Start in staff pose (page 167). Bend both knees, placing the feet flat on the floor then drop your left knee to the floor and step your right foot to the outside of the left thigh, keeping the right foot flat on the floor. On an inhale, raise your left arm to the ceiling. On an exhale, twist to the right. The torso will press against the inside of your right thigh. Place your left elbow to the outside of your right knee keeping the fingertips pointing toward the ceiling. Reach behind your body with the right hand and rest it on the ground for balance. With each inhale twist more deeply into the pose. Never lead the twist with your head. Lead with the heart; your head should be the last part of your body to turn. Inhale to lengthen your spine and rotate farther as you exhale.

Modifications: Sit on a rolled blanket if you're having trouble keeping both sitting bones firmly on the floor. If you have tight hips, keep your bottom leg extended. If it's difficult to place your opposite-side elbow to the outside of your raised leg, hold your front shin with your hand.

SIDE PLANK

VASISTHASANA

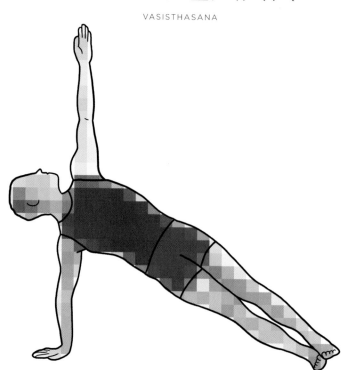

Type of pose: An arm balance and core strengthener.

What it's good for: Strengthens the arms, core, wrists, and legs; improves balance.

Key points: From plank (page 156), slowly roll to the right, bringing your left hand to your left hip. Your supporting hand should be slightly in front of the shoulder, so that your supporting arm is slightly angled relative to the floor. Maintain a microbend in the supporting arm, and push into the floor with your fingertips and the bases of your fingers. Don't let your

hips sag; lift them away from the ground as you push out through the bottoms of your feet. Raise the top arm straight up until it forms a long line with your supporting arm. Your head should be aligned with your spine.

Modifications: If the full pose is too challenging, prop yourself up on your forearm, with your hips stacked. For added support, put your bottom knee on the mat.

Next level: Gaze up toward your hand and raise your top leg, holding it parallel to the floor.

STAFF

DANDASANA

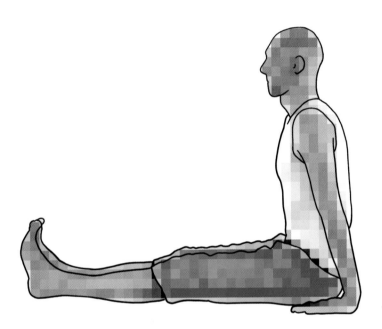

Type of pose: A foundational seated pose.

What it's good for: Improves posture; strengthens the abs and back muscles.

Key points: Sit on the floor with your legs extended out in front of you and your weight on your sitting bones. Flex your feet and press through your heels, strongly engaging your thigh muscles. Place your hands on the floor next to your hips, pressing your palms into the ground with your fingers pointing forward. Keep your spine long.

Modifications: If your hamstrings are tight, sit on a bolster or blanket to keep your spine vertical. It's okay to bend your knees in order to keep your spine straight.

STANDING FORWARD FOLD

UTTANASANA

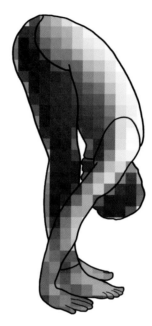

Type of pose: A standing pose with a forward fold and inversion.

What it's good for: Helps relieve stress; stimulates the liver and kidneys; improves digestion; reduces fatigue and anxiety; relieves tension in the neck and shoulders; relieves headaches and insomnia; stretches the hamstrings, calves, and hips; therapeutic for high blood pressure and asthma.

Key points: This pose isn't about touching your toes. Hinge from your hip joints, not from your waist. Think about lengthening the front of your torso as you fold forward, and avoid rounding your back. Keep the tops of your thighs turned slightly inward, and don't lock your knees. The more you engage your quads by drawing them upward, the more your hamstrings will release. Keep the weight in the balls of your feet.

Modifications: If your lower back or hamstrings are tight, bend your knees and let your belly come to your thighs. If the floor seems miles away, place your hands on blocks or cross your forearms and hold your elbows.

Next level: To deepen the stretch, clasp your elbows behind your knees or lock your fingers around your big toes and bend your elbows as you hinge forward.

STANDING HALF FORWARD FOLD

ARDHA UTTANASANA

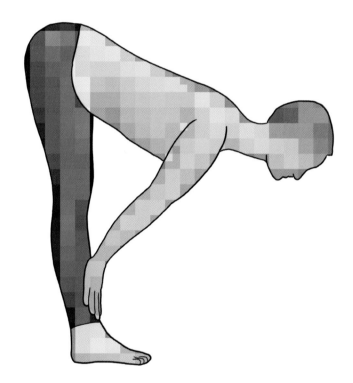

Type of pose: A standing forward fold.

What it's good for: Strengthens the back; improves posture.

Key points: In standing forward fold (page 168), press your fingertips or palms onto the mat beside your feet. As you inhale, straighten your elbows and allow your hands to rise to your shins as you raise your chest, extending forward so you have a slight arch in your back. Look forward, breathe, and on an exhalation, release into standing forward fold.

Modifications: If you can't touch the floor with your hands, bend your knees; alternatively, place your hands on blocks set outside of each foot.

SUPPORTED HEADSTAND

SALAMBA SIRSASANA

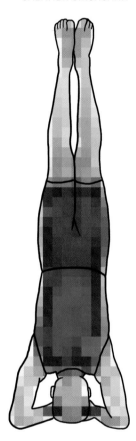

Type of pose: An inversion and balance pose.

What it's good for: Strengthens the arms, legs, and spine; improves digestion; tones the abdominal organs; calms the mind; stimulates the pituitary gland.

Key points: Beginners often take too much weight onto the head and neck, rather than the shoulders and arms, when coming in and out of this pose. Don't kick into the pose; start by tucking your knees up, and then eventually extend your legs into the air. Support the back of your head against clasped hands.

Modifications: Perform the pose against a wall to work on balance.

SUPPORTED SHOULDER STAND

SALAMBA SARVANGASANA

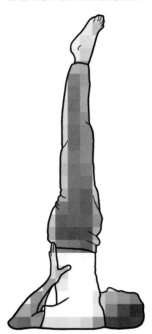

Type of pose: An inversion and balance pose.

What it's good for: Relieves stress and fatigue; improves digestion; stretches the shoulders and neck; stimulates the prostate gland and thyroid.

Key points: Start by lying on your back, knees bent, with the soles of your feet on the floor. On an inhalation, use your abs to lift your legs and hips off the ground, bringing your knees toward your face. Bring your torso perpendicular to the floor by lifting your hips. Bend your elbows and place your hands on your lower back for support. Avoid letting your elbows splay out to the sides, and don't let your upper arms roll inward. Spread both palms wide against the back of your torso. Try to bring your shoulders, elbows, and hips into one line. Straighten your legs and reach your feet toward the ceiling. Keep your head and neck in line with your spine, and don't turn your head side to side.

Modifications: To protect your neck, place a folded blanket beneath your shoulders before coming into the pose; your head and neck should be off the blanket. Start by lifting one leg at a time.

TABLE

BHARMANASANA

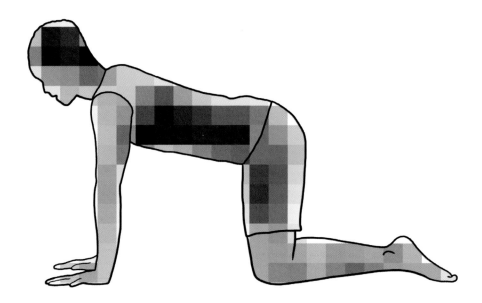

Type of pose: A foundational pose and transitional posture.

What it's good for: Builds core strength; lengthens the spine; improves posture and balance.

Key points: Your knees should be hip-width apart, with your feet directly behind your knees. Your palms should be directly under your shoulders. Keep your back flat and gaze forward just ahead of your hands.

Modifications: If you have sensitive wrists or knees, use a blanket for extra cushioning.

Next level: Challenge your balance by raising the opposite arm and leg parallel to the floor.

TREE

VRKSASANA

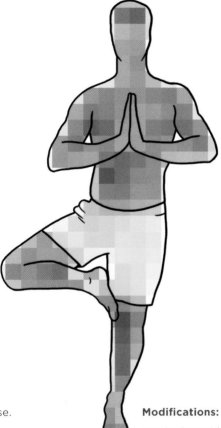

Type of pose: A standing balance pose.

What it's good for: Strengthens the thighs, calves, ankles, and spine; stretches the inner thighs, groin, chest, and shoulders; improves balance and concentration; therapeutic for sciatica and flat feet.

Key points: Never rest your foot on your knee; always place it above or below the knee. Keep your hips square.

Modifications: If you can't bring your foot to your thigh, rest it alongside the calf or ankle of the standing leg. You can stand with your back against a wall if you feel unsteady.

Next level: Closing your eyes will increase the challenge of maintaining your balance.

UPWARD DOG

URDHVA MUKHA SVANASANA

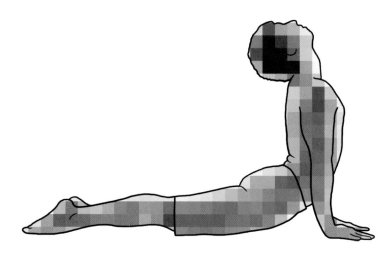

Type of pose: A heart opener, backbend and transitional pose.

What it's good for: Strengthens the spine, arms, and wrists; improves posture; stretches the chest, shoulders, and abdomen; helps relieve fatigue and sciatica.

Key points: Proper hand placement is key. Start by lying facedown with your hands next to your lower ribs. As you lift up, avoid collapsing into your shoulders. Actively draw your shoulders away from your ears by pulling your

shoulder blades toward your tailbone. You want the sides of your ribs, not the front of your ribs, to push forward; this prevents putting pressure on the lower back. Look straight ahead or extend your head back slightly. The tops of your feet should push firmly into the mat to lift your legs, knees, and pelvis off the ground. Try not to grip your glutes.

Modifications: If you're having trouble keeping your legs suspended, place a rolled blanket below the tops of your thighs before you move into the pose. Rest your thighs on the blanket as you press your tailbone down.

UPWARD SALUTE

URDHVA HASTASANA

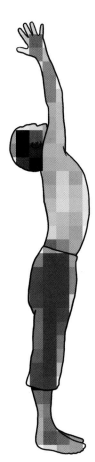

Type of pose: A standing pose and mild backbend.

What it's good for: Stretches the shoulders; improves digestion; alleviates back pain.

Key points: In mountain pose (page 154) rotate your arms outward to face your palms forward and, on an inhalation, sweep your arms out to the sides and up toward the ceiling. Press your hands together, tip your head back slightly, and gaze at your thumbs.

Modifications: If you have tight shoulders, leave your arms parallel above your head, rather than touching your hands together.

WARRIOR 1

VIRABHADRASANA 1

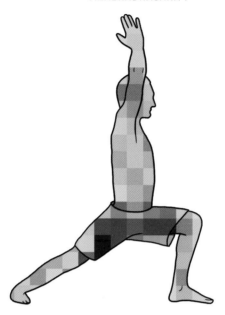

Type of pose: A standing and strengthening pose.

What it's good for: Stretches the chest, shoulders, neck, and psoas; strengthens the shoulders, arms, and back; stretches and strengthens the thighs, calves, and arches of the feet; soothes sciatica; improves concentration.

Key points: From mountain pose (page 154), step one foot back four to five feet. The toes of your front foot should point toward the top of the mat. Pivot your back foot outward at a 45-degree angle. Your front heel should be aligned with the arch of your back foot. Keep your pelvis turned toward the front of the mat; you can place your

hands on your hips to check alignment. Ground down with the outer edge of the back foot, keeping your back leg straight. As you bend your front knee to 90 degrees, avoid tipping your pelvis forward, as that would compress the lower back. Instead, lift up through your chest and lengthen your tailbone toward the floor.

Modifications: If you have trouble keeping your back heel grounded and your lower back lengthened, rest your back heel on a blanket. If you have tight hips, try doing the pose with heel-to-heel alignment, rather than heel-to-arch. This will give you more room to square your hips.

WARRIOR 2

VIRABHADRASANA 2

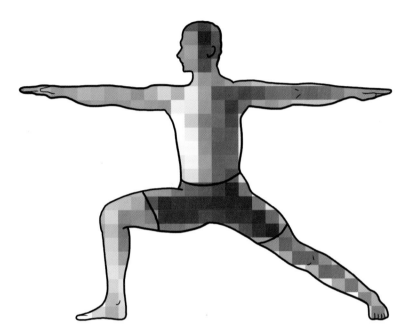

Type of pose: A hip opener and standing and strengthening pose.

What it's good for: Strengthens and stretches the legs and ankles; stretches the groins, chest, lungs, and shoulders; increases stamina and concentration; therapeutic for back pain, sciatica, and flat feet.

Key points: From warrior I (page 176) bring your arms down and out to the sides as you turn your torso to face the long edge of the mat. Be mindful that your front knee doesn't drift inward; this will strain the knee joint. Keep it aligned with the front ankle, your lower leg perpendicular to the floor. Stay strong in your back leg, pressing the outer back heel firmly to the floor with your back foot at a 45-degree angle. Maintain heel-to-heel alignment. Don't lean your torso over your front thigh. Reach wide, from fingertip to fingertip, while allowing your shoulders to drop and lifting your chest. Gaze out toward your front fingers.

Modifications: If you have tight hips, shorten your stance. You can also perform this pose against a wall to work on alignment and to keep your front knee from drifting inward.

WARRIOR 3

VIRABHADRASANA 3

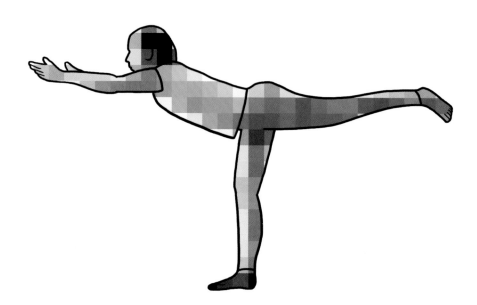

Type of pose: A standing balance and strengthening pose.

What it's good for: Improves balance, posture, and concentration; strengthens the ankles, hamstrings, shoulders, back, and abdomen.

Key points: Start from a high lunge position. Bend your torso forward to just above your front thigh and keep your hands on your hips or stretch your arms forward. As you straighten your front knee, firm up the quad of the standing leg, pressing the head of the thighbone back.

This centers the femur in the hip joint. As your standing leg straightens, lift your back leg. You ultimately want your body to look like a T shape from the side, with your arms, torso, and back leg parallel to the floor. Avoid putting most of your weight into the standing hip and hyperextending the standing knee.

Modifications: If you have trouble balancing, try resting your hands gently against a wall.

Next level: Enter the pose from warrior 1 (page 176), with your arms stretched upward.

WIDE-ANGLE SEATED FORWARD FOLD

UPAVISTHA KONASANA

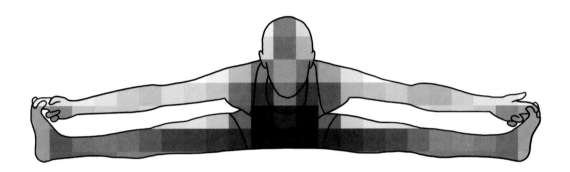

Type of pose: A seated forward fold and hip opener.

What it's good for: Detoxes the kidneys; therapeutic for arthritis and sciatica; stimulates the abdominal organs; strengthens the spine; stretches the hamstrings and groins; calms the mind; improves digestion.

Key points: Your kneecaps should point toward the ceiling. Keep your leg muscles engaged and don't lock your knees. Fold from your hips, not your waist, to avoid rounding your spine.

Modifications: If you have tight hamstrings, bend your knees or place rolled blankets beneath your knees. If your torso doesn't touch the ground, rest it on a bolster or rolled blanket in front of you.

Next level: Wrap your fingers around your big toes and pull back on your toes, bending your elbows out to the sides as you lean forward.

WIDE-LEGGED FORWARD FOLD

PRASARITA PADOTTANASANAT

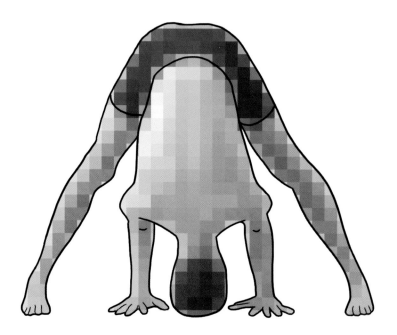

Type of pose: A standing forward fold, a hip opener and a mild inversion.

What it's good for: Alleviates headaches, fatigue, and backache; calms the mind; strengthens and stretches the hamstrings and spine; stretches the hips.

Key points: Turn your toes slightly inward and keep your feet engaged. Lift your inner arches by drawing your inner ankles up, and press the outer edges of your feet and the balls of your big toes into the floor. Fold from the hips

and concentrate on lengthening your torso rather than rounding your spine. Don't lock your knees.

Modifications: Most beginners can't touch their head, or even their hands, to the floor. If that's you, use a block, bolster, or blanket to support your head or hands.

Next level: Once your hands comfortably touch the ground, try interlacing your fingers behind your back and extending your knuckles overhead as you fold.

WIDE SQUAT

MALASANA

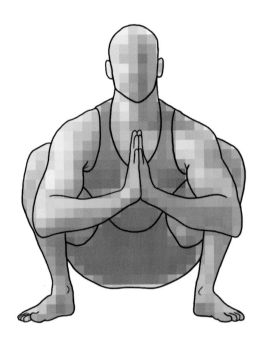

Type of pose: A standing pose and hip opener.

What it's good for: Improves digestion; calms the mind; stretches the ankles, groins, and back of the torso; increases circulation and blood flow in the pelvis, which can help increase sex drive.

Key points: Lengthen the front of your torso by pressing your elbows against your inner knees. Keep your weight in your heels. Don't bounce your hips.

Modifications: If your heels come off the floor, support them on a folded mat or blanket. If you have trouble balancing, rest your sitting bones on a block until you gain enough strength to stay elevated.

Next level: Press your inner thighs against the sides of your torso and extend your arms forward and out to the sides until your shins are in your armpits. Press your fingertips to the floor or clasp the back of your heels.

INDEX

ACKNOWLEDGMENTS

I believe the teacher is just as important as the breath. Over time, a good teacher can peel back the layers of yoga and all of its benefits. I've been lucky to have practiced with incredibly fun, knowledgeable, free-spirited instructors. Thanks and endless gratitude to Andrea Maltzer, April Puciata, Erica Gragg, David Magone, Jayne Gottlieb, Rusty Wells, and Nicole Cronin, as well as Kelly Elle Kenworthy and Amy Benton of the Little Yoga Studio in Boulder, Colorado, my local studio. Enormous thanks to Andrew Tanner for championing this book. And toWv my fellow yogini, Leanne Arcuri, for offering encouragement throughout multiple drafts. Much gratitude to Nick Fauchald and the team at Dovetail for believing that I had this book in me. I have to thank the team at Wanderlust—Chad Dennis, Sean Hoess, and Jeff Krasno—for supporting this book. Their festivals have introduced yoga to an entirely new audience and have made yoga more about a healthy lifestyle than a trendy workout or spiritual practice. Most of all, thanks to my guy friends for sharing stories (even the embarrassing ones) and for making time to talk with me while trying to juggle work, family, the gym...and a few minutes a day for yoga.

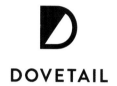

DOVETAIL

Text copyright © 2017 by Jen Murphy

Design and illustrations by Will Pay

Published by Dovetail Press in Brooklyn, New York, a division of Assembly Brands LLC.

For details or ordering information, contact the publisher at the address below or email **info@dovetail.press**.

Dovetail Press

42 West Street #403

Brooklyn, NY 11222

www.dovetail.press

Library of Congress Cataloging-in-Publication data is on file with the publisher.

ISBN: 978-0-9898882-5-7

First Edition

Printed in the United States

10 9 8 7 6 5 4 3 2 1